MS & ME

Living a full life beyond diagnosis, with a resilient mindset and an anti-inflammatory lifestyle

Laura Lamont

MS & ME

© Copyright 2024. Laura Lamont

All Rights Reserved. No part of this publication may be reproduced, distributed, or transmitted in any form or by any means, including photocopying, recording, or other electronic or mechanical methods, without the publisher's prior written permission.

Table of Contents

Introduction 4

Chapter 1 13

Where It All Began For Me 13

Chapter 2 25

Down South 25

Chapter 3 36

City Life 36

Chapter 4 42

A Period of Settling 42

Chapter 5 48

The Diagnosis 48

Chapter 6 56

A woman's home is Her Mansion 56

Chapter 7 63

Anyone for coffee 63

Chapter 8 72

The Dawn of a New Beginning 72

Chapter 9 75

A Time for A New Beginning 75

Chapter 10 84

Over to You 84

MS & ME

Introduction

Setting the Stage

From Pneumonia to Purpose: A Journey with MS

Here I stand at 61 and three-quarters! It's astonishing how quickly the years have flown by, seemingly in the blink of an eye. Officially, I'm in the enviable position of early retirement, though I don't quite feel retired at all. I've embarked on an entirely new adventure: writing and publishing self-help books. And beyond that, I've got a couple of novels tucked away, waiting to be brought to life, not to mention this very book—ms and ME.

This book is personal to me and my own M.S. journey, and I sincerely hope it demonstrates to others, particularly the newly diagnosed, that *life does not end with a diagnosis—it transforms.* While the path may be uncertain and challenging, it can also be filled with strength, growth, and unexpected joys. I want this book to be a source of hope, showing that with the right mindset, support, and determination, it is possible to live a fulfilling, vibrant, and meaningful life, no matter what obstacles M.S. may place in your way. *You are not alone, and it's that old cliché! you are stronger than you think.*

In 2022, we made a significant life change, leaving behind our long-time family home in Bristol to settle in a small, peaceful town along the southern coast of Scotland. This marks the beginning of a new chapter for us, perhaps even our swan song. You might wonder why we made such a bold move. The answer is simple: to truly enjoy life in a serene and beautiful area, far removed from the hustle and bustle of our former city. Plus, the considerably lower cost of housing here meant we could free up funds, allowing us to live the lifestyle we've always dreamed of, with greater financial ease and freedom.

After years of living in a whirlwind of busyness, business, and chaos, I've relished the opportunity to slow down and appreciate a more relaxed pace. However, I'm the kind of person who thrives on having a project to sink my teeth into. While I've enjoyed the calm, I've never been one to sit idle for too long. Over the past two years, I've dipped my toes into various business ventures, exploring different avenues, yet somehow, they didn't quite ignite my passion the way I'd hoped. On a positive note, they certainly have not been a waste of my time the health products I have discovered during my investigations have benefited my health! I will talk about them later.

And then, I found myself here—in this deeply rewarding space—creating books designed to help others. Writing has given me purpose, a new sense of direction, and a way to channel my energy into something meaningful. It's a new adventure, an extension of my Life Coaching that doesn't tie me to weekly meetings with clients. One that allows me to continue growing, learning, and contributing, during this stage of life. And it feels like exactly where I'm meant to be. This book isn't going to be about the nitty-gritty of every part of my life, loves found and lost etc, etc but more about my health and well-being on my way to where I am today.

Recent statistics show that MS affects over 2.8 million people worldwide, with women outnumbering men nearly 4 to 1. When I received my diagnosis, these numbers weren't as well documented, and the treatment options were far more limited. Today, research has expanded dramatically, and our understanding of autoimmune conditions has evolved significantly.

What you'll find in these pages is my journey with MS, but more importantly, you'll discover how this condition became an unexpected teacher, pushing me to understand the profound connection between mind, body, and spirit. Each chapter will explore different phases of my life, from the early warning signs to my current approach to managing health and wellness.

Throughout this book, I'll share not just my personal experiences, but also the latest medical insights and research that have helped shape my understanding of MS. You'll find practical advice about diet, lifestyle changes, and the importance of maintaining a positive outlook, all while navigating the very real challenges that come with an autoimmune condition.

(Health Context: An autoimmune disease occurs when the body's immune system mistakenly attacks its own healthy cells, tissues, or organs, believing them to be foreign invaders. Instead of protecting the body from harmful pathogens, the immune system causes inflammation and damage to the body's own tissues. Examples of autoimmune diseases include multiple sclerosis, rheumatoid arthritis, lupus, Fibromyalgia, and type 1 diabetes.)

When I received my diagnosis, it wasn't entirely a shock. My sister, who is five years older than I am, had been diagnosed with the exact same condition at the same age. It's almost surreal, isn't it? You start to wonder if it's in the family genes. Our great uncle, who lived in Aberdeen, also had MS. I remember hearing stories of how he spent many years wheelchair-bound, battling the disease. But I'm not going to dwell too much on his, or my sister's story—that's hers to tell. Sadly, though, she has followed a path all too similar to our great uncle's. So, despite our identical gene pool my story is one of Joy and hope for others and I really hope that you will follow a similar path to me.

[Health History Context: Research indicates that having a first-degree relative with MS increases one's risk of developing the condition. However, the disease's progression can vary significantly

MS & ME

even among family members, suggesting that lifestyle factors play a crucial role.]

What struck me as odd during early M.S. episodes was that no one actually said to me, outright, "You have multiple sclerosis." I understand that it is a condition that is often diagnosed retrospectively but there was this uncomfortable avoidance of directly naming the illness. At the time, I was working as a teacher when suddenly, I lost the use of my right side, and my vision doubled, for three months I was unable to function properly. The guilt of being absent from my teaching position weighed heavily on me—I felt like I was letting everyone down, my family, my students, and my colleagues alike. I even remember phoning my union, hoping for some guidance, some form of assistance, but all I got was a disheartening dismissal. They offered no help at all, leaving me feeling even more lost. I found myself wondering, "How will our young family cope if I'm no longer able to work? How will we survive?"

It wasn't just about losing my income; the timing of it all seemed tragically ironic. We had already been through several turbulent years, with me in university pursuing my degree. When I started my B.Ed. Hons, we had one child—our almost five-year-old son. By the time I finished four years later, we had three children. Some might call that bad planning! Finances were always tight, especially after my partner was made redundant and had to take a job that paid significantly less. Suddenly, here we were, with three young children, and I had become the primary earner. And now, in the midst of all this, I was seriously unwell, each day wondering if I would ever recover enough to return to work, to be the mother and partner my family needed.

In the back of my mind, I kept recalling my sister's experience with relapsing-remitting MS. Her journey, at that stage, had informed me that this might pass, that it was possible I would regain my strength and function. But even with that knowledge, I couldn't help but feel an overwhelming sense of uncertainty. Each day was a struggle to balance hope with the reality of our situation, and it was scary not knowing what the future held for me and my family.

What could have been a deeply distressing three months turned out to be a period of surprising resilience and family unity. I was fortunate enough to be able to return to my job after those three months, which, in retrospect, now feels like a relatively short time. My husband, despite the uncertainty, managed to secure work with his previous employer again, even though it was agency work at the time. Their support was invaluable—they allowed him the flexibility to dart in and out of work to drop off and pick up the children from school, ensuring that our home life ran as smoothly as possible amidst the chaos.

But still, I was grateful. Grateful that it was "only" three months, and that afterward, I was able to resume my position at work. I knew, though, that things would never be quite the same. I had been ambitious, and eager to climb the career ladder and take on more responsibilities, but this experience changed my perspective. I realized that in my line of work, the demands of the job were already heavy enough without adding extra layers of responsibility. With a heavy heart, I had to relinquish the additional duties I had once embraced so enthusiastically. It wasn't easy to step back, but I knew I had to, for the sake of my health and my family.

Thankfully, my employer was as supportive as my husband had been. They understood the situation and were kind enough to accommodate my needs without question, which was an enormous relief. We had no close family members nearby to help us, and unfortunately, my partner's family never reached out to lend a hand. It was just us—our little unit—navigating through this challenging time. But we didn't let it overwhelm us or diminish our spirit. We didn't allow the difficulties to define our family life.

In fact, we even managed to take the children on an Easter holiday to North Wales. It was such a memorable trip—we hiked up Snowdon, and although we couldn't hike all the way to the summit, we went on the train, we did walk the last few hundred meters. I remember how fierce the wind was up there; it was so strong that I had to hold on to our youngest for dear life as we ascended. At one point, our eldest got caught by a powerful gust of wind and was nearly swept away, but I managed to grab him just in time before disaster could strike. Looking back now, it feels almost surreal, but moments like that have a way of staying with you—both the fear and the exhilaration of coming through it all unscathed.

When I reflect on that period, what stands out the most isn't the worry or the hardships. Instead, I remember the moments of love and tenderness, like sitting on the sofa with my two youngest children, my "university babies," as they showered my face with kisses, playfully competing over who loved me more. Those small, precious moments carried me through. Our eldest, too, really rose to the occasion. Whenever his dad was at work, he would step in and take on the little, yet essential tasks, like making me a cup of tea, showing a level of maturity far beyond his years.

In the midst of what could have been a dark time, my family became a source of strength and joy. Those three months taught me more about resilience, love, and the importance of cherishing the good, even when life seems to throw its worst at you.

We decided to seek out a private MS specialist, hoping to gain more insight and guidance beyond what we had encountered so far. The consultation was eye-opening in ways I hadn't anticipated. It was during this visit that I first became aware of the profound importance of diet in managing MS. The specialist recommended a "Stone Age" or paleo-style diet—essentially a regimen based on what our ancestors would have eaten in prehistoric times, long before modern processed foods took over. He emphasized that diet could play a crucial role in managing my symptoms and improving my overall health.

At the time, however, implementing such a diet wasn't as simple as it sounds. With young children to feed and a family to manage, it felt almost impossible to fully embrace this lifestyle change. On top of that, organic food was incredibly hard to come by in those days—if you did manage to find it, it was outrageously expensive. Organic options were practically non-existent for ordinary families; they were more the preserve of the very well-off. Nonetheless, the core principles of that consultation stayed with us. We made small adjustments where we could, and even though we couldn't fully commit to the "Stone Age" diet back then, the idea of clean, whole foods became a lasting theme in our lives.

Over time, this dietary philosophy evolved into something we could more easily adopt. These days, we follow a largely organic, whole-food-based diet—well, 90% of the time at least. I must admit, I still can't resist the occasional packet of crisps or a bit of chocolate! But compared to where we were back then, we're much closer to what that specialist originally advised. Looking back, I really appreciate the advice he gave, even though I couldn't afford to go back for follow-up consultations. At the time, it felt like I was being handed this valuable key to better health, but the financial realities meant that we had to figure out the journey on our own.

Now, it's so much easier to follow his guidelines. The availability of organic produce, the variety of foods, and even the knowledge surrounding gut health and autoimmune conditions have all expanded. What I've learned along the way is that it's not about perfection but about making the best possible choices consistently.

For example, I've found that with organic meat, the quality is so much better that you don't need as much to feel satisfied, so it balances out the cost in the end. If you've never tried it, I highly recommend giving it a go—you may find that you need less, and the difference in taste and nutrition is well worth it.

I came across an interesting statistic recently: if the entire global population were to switch to organic diets, 30% of people could die from starvation due to food shortages. This really struck me, as it reminded me just how privileged we are to have access to such high-quality, nutrient-dense foods here in this country. It also brought home how lucky I am to be in a position where I can make these choices for my health. But it's not just about me and my MS—this understanding of diet and gut health extends far beyond my own condition.

I truly believe that the same principles of nutrition apply to anyone suffering from an autoimmune illness. There's a reason people refer to the gut as our "second brain." The food we eat has a direct impact on how we feel, both physically and mentally. The old sayings, like "Let food be thy medicine," ring truer than ever for me. Over the years, I've come to realize that these aren't just clichés—they hold real wisdom. Whether you're managing a chronic illness or simply trying to maintain good health, the power of diet should never be underestimated. The connection between what we eat and how we live is undeniable, and I feel fortunate to have been guided toward this knowledge, even if the journey wasn't easy at first.

With all of this in mind, I come to the conclusion of this introduction. I want to leave you with a deep conviction that has become a guiding principle in my life: what we choose to nourish our bodies and our minds with, has a profound and undeniable impact on both our physical and mental well-being. Our diet influences not just our energy and vitality, but also our ability to face life's challenges with strength and resilience. The food we eat has the potential to either sustain or undermine our health, and I firmly believe that by making conscious choices, we can give ourselves the best chance to live a long, healthy, and fulfilling life.

Now that I've set the stage and shared the core beliefs that have shaped my path, it's time to dive into the story itself—the journey that brought me here, the lessons learned along the way, and the experiences that I hope will inspire and empower others. So, without further ado, let's begin.

*[**Key Takeaway:** The foundations of health are laid early in life, but our ability to influence our well-being continues throughout our journey. My story demonstrates that while we may inherit certain predispositions, our lifestyle choices and responses to challenges play a crucial role in determining our health outcomes.]*

Chapter 1

Where It All Began For Me

I was born in the notorious winter of 1962/63, the coldest winter on record. Rotten Row (what a name!) Maternity Hospital in Glasgow was the place where my life began. The third child of my parents and the third caesarean section for my mother. My lungs were as cold as the weather, I was born with pneumonia and remained in hospital alone in an incubator for several weeks. This was the start of a turbulent year for the whole family, my-grandmother, my brother, and my sister had to go to school in the city for several months to keep the family supported by our nana and great-grandmother. I have a dent in my left leg, where the medical interventions kept me alive. My earliest memory was probably an early childhood dream where my nana and great aunt Meg stood over my incubator expressing their concern for "the poor wee lamb". It's a family myth that my aversion to hugs is due to my time untouched in that incubator. Maybe there is some underlying resentment for the abandonment as I really don't have a problem hugging people beyond my parents and siblings.

Obviously, I recovered, as I am still here! Until I was around five, I could make the most horrendous rasping noises when I got out of breath, beyond that I made a full recovery. At the time of my birth, my family was living in a very damp seaside ex-school house that the Scottish Education Department had allotted to my father when he was sent to an Art teaching Job in a school in the most Southern West town of Scotland. As you can tell from this, geographically I have moved full circle to where my life began. It was just over a year after my birth that the family moved into town to a newly built house with heating and windows that didn't drip with condensation and damp walls. I was often jealous that I didn't get to live long at the school house as my older siblings aged around 7 and 6 when we moved used to have great fun regularly breaking into the abandoned school that was attached to our house and playing teacher and pupils, with all the teaching materials left, this "Marie Celeste" old school was a fabulous playground.

[Reflection: Environmental factors are now known to play a crucial role in autoimmune conditions. The combination of damp living conditions and my early respiratory challenges may have contributed to my immune system's later responses.]

We only lived in the new building for a couple of years. My only memory is of my brother stealing my lovely red peddle car and hurtling down the hill by our house and crashing into the wall. I don't know whether he was hurt or not all I cared about was my shiny car. Years later I was told by a clairvoyant never to buy a red car, I think she was about 40 years too late! So off we all went, leaving the warm and cozy new build and off to a drafty old farmhouse.

The farmhouse is a mere field away from the comfort of modernity, yet worlds apart in terms of living conditions. It marked the start of another chapter, a different kind of life where the luxuries of warmth and convenience gave way to the more rustic charm of the countryside. But as with everything, we adapted, and that farmhouse became the backdrop for the next phase of our family's journey.

The three-story farmhouse, with all its faded grandeur, was an enchanting place during the day. It boasted vast, high-ceilinged rooms that seemed to stretch on forever, and in the kitchen, a charming old yellow Aga stood as the heart of the home. My mum used to love to sit on the closed lids of the Aga and drink Ideal Milk, probably a contribution to her diagnosis of Diabetes years later! That Aga was soon replaced by a shiny blue oil-fired version, but I'll always remember the warmth and comfort the old one brought to our lives. By day, the house was full of light and life, a perfect playground for imaginative children like myself and my siblings. The sheer size of the rooms gave us endless possibilities for games, and there was always something about the history of the place that made it feel both special and a little mysterious.

But when night fell, the house took on a very different character, especially for me as a young child. What had felt grand and fun in the daylight became eerie and unsettling in the dark. My bedroom was situated on the top floor, while the rest of the family would often be two storeys down. The isolation was terrifying at times. I remember lying in bed, listening to the creaks and groans of the old house, convinced that something or someone was lurking in the shadows. It was a spooky house, full of strange noises and long, dark hallways that, to a child, seemed to stretch on forever. Being sent to bed alone up there felt like a nightly ordeal, my imagination running wild as I lay awake, too scared to sleep.

Still, despite its spookiness, the house had plenty of redeeming qualities. I have fond memories of playing on the half-landing where a large wicker chest sat, a relic of another time. My siblings and I would spend hours there, re-enacting scenes from the children's show "Andy Pandy," which those, of a certain age, who grew up in the UK will surely remember from "Watch With Mother." The show featured Andy, Teddy, and Looby Loo, though there was always some debate about whether Andy was a boy or a girl. In our games, I was always cast as Looby Loo, but much to my dismay, I was never allowed inside the wicker basket like Andy and Teddy. Instead, I had to lie on the stairs, watching my siblings as they took the starring roles. It was an odd game, to be sure, but it filled many happy afternoons in that quirky old house.

One of the most intriguing discoveries during our time there came courtesy of my brother, who was always the curious meddler. One day, while the whole family was gathered in the ground-floor family room, he began poking around in one of the cupboards. After noticing that the back of the cupboard sounded hollow, his natural instinct was to investigate further. Before we knew it, he had bashed a hole through the back of the cupboard, revealing something none of us had ever imagined—a hidden set of steps descending deep into the ground.

We were all astonished as we realized that beneath our very home lay a secret tunnel that stretched several meters underground. It turned out that this tunnel had been there for decades, possibly even longer, and had served as a shelter during the World Wars. At one time, there had been a full room at the end of the tunnel, but later owners had sealed it off, leaving only the mysterious steps and the dark passageway that seemed to disappear into the earth.

For us children, that tunnel became both a source of fascination and terror. It sparked countless adventures and tales of hidden treasures or wartime secrets, but it also added to the already spooky atmosphere of the house. Every time we played near the tunnel, there was a sense of thrill mixed with fear, as if we were stepping into the unknown. It became yet another layer in the complex and intriguing world of that old farmhouse, a place that seemed to hold more stories than we could ever uncover during our time there.

Looking back, I realize that the farmhouse was far more than just a place to live. It was a backdrop to our childhood, a stage on which countless memories, both magical and frightening, were made. The grandeur, the spookiness, and the mystery all combined to create an environment that shaped who we were as children, and who we would become as adults. It was a place where imagination ran wild, and where every corner, every cupboard, and every shadow seemed to have a story of its own.

Those years in the farmhouse were not only marked by the eerie atmosphere of the house or the thrill of childhood discoveries but also by a deep undercurrent of sadness and distress that had nothing to do with the house itself. Unfortunately, much of the turmoil in those years was tied to my father's mental health, something that cast a long shadow over our family life. As children, we didn't fully understand the complexities of what he was going through, but we certainly bore the brunt of it. The violence that occurred during this time left scars, especially for my brother, the eldest, who seemed to clash with our father more than anyone else. Their relationship was particularly volatile, and many of their interactions were fraught with tension and anger. The clashes were frequent, intense, and often frightening for the rest of the family of us to witness.

But it wasn't just my brother who found himself at the mercy of our father's moods. My sister, and occasionally even I, would feel the sting of his rage. Looking back on it now, as an adult, I can understand that my father was a tormented soul, a man haunted by his own past. He had been a victim of his own father's brutality, and that pain manifested in his interactions with us. He was, in many ways, trapped—an incredibly creative person stuck in a job that drained him, teaching in an environment he despised. His frustrations and unhappiness boiled over at home, often in cruel and cutting ways.

I can still hear him shouting, the words etched into my memory: "I put up with little bastards all day, and then I have to come home to you little bastards!" His anger would escalate, and sometimes, in moments of even deeper frustration, he would yell, "You are nothing." Those words cut the deepest, and even now, decades later, I can't bear to hear anyone say that to another person. The idea that someone could be reduced to "nothing" is unbearable to me because I know how damaging those words can be. No one should ever feel like they're "nothing."

Of course, as children, we didn't just hear the anger; we also absorbed the lessons from his outbursts. I learned more than my fair share of colourful swear words from my father during those years. But beyond the language, it was the fear that stuck with me. As a small child, he was terrifying. The unpredictability of his temper created an environment where we were constantly on edge, never quite knowing when things would erupt. There was a distinct pattern to his behaviour, though, one that we came to recognize over time. During the school term, when the pressures of his job were weighing on him, life at home was hell. But once school holidays arrived, and the demands of his work were lifted, he became a different person altogether—lighter, more relaxed, even fun to be around. I now understand my dislike of men in formal suits, dad hated wearing suits and ties but had to for work, when he wasn't wearing that suit, he was the relaxed and authentic version of dad that we loved!

It was a strange duality to live with, this oscillation between fear and enjoyment. During the holidays, we would experience the best of him. He could be playful, often charming, and we'd have moments of real family fun. But those periods of reprieve only served to highlight the darkness of the school terms when the anger and frustration returned, and our home became a battleground once more.

As I reflect on those years, I now see my father in a more nuanced light. He wasn't just the frightening figure I remember from my childhood; he was a deeply troubled man, struggling with his own demons and trapped in a life that didn't fulfil him. He was an artist, stifled by a job that offered him no outlet for his own creativity, and that frustration consumed him. It doesn't excuse the violence or the hurtful words, but it does help me understand him better now. And to his credit, as we all grew older, my father made efforts to make peace with us. He reached out in his own way, trying to heal the wounds he had inflicted, and we found reconciliation.

Still, the scars of those years run deep. The fear, the volatility, and the sadness of watching someone you love wrestle with their own pain while inadvertently causing you harm is not something you easily forget. The memories of that time, the swings between terror and joy, remain a complicated part of my past, shaping who I am today. In the end, my father was neither a monster nor a saint, but a man deeply flawed and deeply human, navigating his own struggles in a way that profoundly affected those around him.

[Reflection: The impact of stress and trauma on physical health is now well-documented. Witnessing my father's struggles helped me understand the importance of managing both mental and physical well-being in maintaining overall health.]

In addition to our parents, our nana—my mum's mother—played a pivotal role in our upbringing. She became a constant presence in our lives, particularly when she moved into a mobile home in our garden after being forced to sell her beloved bungalow. That bungalow had been where she lived with Munner, our great-grandmother. After Munner passed away—an event I distinctly recall happening during an episode of *The Virginian*, though my mother disputes this memory—Nana found herself in a difficult position. Her extremely wealthy brother-in-law, who had contributed money toward the bungalow's purchase, pressured her into selling it after Munner's death. With nowhere else to go, Nana moved into a mobile home on our property. From that point on, she became a surrogate caregiver for us kids, especially when my mother returned to education to train as a teacher.

It was Nana who was there for me most days when I walked home from school at lunchtime. I can still vividly recall her making me my regular lunches—Scotch Pie with baked beans or, on colder days, a bowl of tomato soup loaded with chunks of white bread. Admittedly, cooking was not a forte for Nana's, but that never seemed to matter. Those simple meals, shared in her cozy mobile home, are some of my fondest memories. Despite her lack of culinary skills, Nana brought so much else into our lives. She had a way of making ordinary moments feel special.

Nana was also the one who indulged us in the world of fashion, buying us the most fashionable clothes. She was a little rebellious in her own right, letting us watch TV shows that were strictly banned by our parents, and teaching us how to play poker—yes, poker! As we grew older, she became even more of a confidante. I remember how she'd secretly share cigarettes with us, creating a sense of trust and sanctuary that we didn't always feel at home. Her mantra "I never inhale you know!" She was our safe harbour in a household that could feel stormy.

[Health Context: Recent studies have shown that emotional support and stress reduction can significantly impact autoimmune conditions. The contrasting environments between our main house and my grandmother's mobile home might have provided early lessons in how the environment affects well-being.]

When my mum went to Teacher Training College, I started school early as a result. I began Primary One in January 1966, when I had just turned just four years old. It was the norm in those days for a small child to walk to and from school even at lunchtime, as I did, it seems unthinkable by modern standards. A few months ago, I retraced that walk, and while it wasn't as far as I had remembered, it still made me reflect on how much times have changed. Back then, parents weren't as consumed by fear. Today, we live with an overwhelming sense of anxiety for our children's safety.

Starting school early came with its own set of challenges. My mother, in her eagerness to succeed at Teacher Training College, used me as something of a project for her coursework. She taught me to read and write well before I started school, thinking it would give me an advantage. However, this was not received well by my Primary One teacher, a stern and bitter woman who resented the fact that I already had these skills. Rather than being praised, I was punished for being ahead of my peers. The teacher's disdain was palpable, and it made my first year at school a far cry from the joyful experience my mother had likely imagined.

As a trained teacher myself, I now understand the complexities of early childhood education in a way that perhaps my mother did not. I don't approve of what she did, despite her good intentions. I believe in the educational philosophy that children are not ready to learn to read until they are around seven years old or, as some theories suggest, when they begin to lose their baby teeth. There is a natural readiness that occurs at that age, and to push children too soon can be detrimental to their development. My own experience in Primary One serves as a reminder of the importance of respecting a child's natural progression, rather than imposing adult expectations too early.

[Reflection: Early childhood stress, whether academic or emotional, is now recognized as a potential trigger for future health conditions. The pressure to perform beyond my developmental stage may have contributed to patterns of stress that would follow me into adulthood.]

In reflecting on these early years, it's clear that nana was an anchor for us during a tumultuous time, offering support and love in ways my parents often couldn't. She may not have been perfect, but her presence in our lives was invaluable. She was the one who provided stability and affection when we needed it most, and for that, I will always be grateful.

Growing up on a farm, to my mind, is one of the most magical experiences a child could have. It provided an endless playground of adventure, imagination, and freedom. My siblings and I spent countless hours exploring the fields, splashing through the burns (small streams), and building forts with fence posts that were neatly stacked in the farm yard. Every day was an adventure, and the farm became our kingdom. We created elaborate games, waged imaginary battles, and found joy in the simplest of things—whether it was chasing each other through the tall grasses or climbing trees in the far-off corners of the fields.

[Health Context: Current research emphasizes the importance of early exposure to natural environments in developing a balanced immune system. The "hygiene hypothesis" suggests that some modern autoimmune conditions may be linked to insufficient early exposure to diverse environmental factors.]

In addition to the sprawling farm, we were fortunate enough to live just a short walk from both the beach and the town. My best friend lived on her parent's farm just up the hill from us. On any given day, we could swap between the countryside and the coast, running through the fields one moment and feeling the sand between our toes the next. It was the kind of childhood where freedom felt boundless, and the world was full of possibilities. In hindsight, I think my dad might have been right when he referred to us as "little bastards," but not in the way he meant it. My parents, though strict in principle, knew little of our actual exploits. While they set many rules, their busy social lives often meant they weren't around to enforce them, and we took full advantage of that freedom.

MS & ME

My parents were social butterflies. If they weren't hosting parties at our house, they were off at one of their friends' homes, enjoying themselves. This left us kids to our own devices more often than not. We were given strict rules, of course, but their frequent absence gave us plenty of room to bend, break, and outright ignore those rules. For example, we were expressly forbidden from going to "the Shows"—the local funfair. But naturally, we went anyway, thrilled by the forbidden excitement of the rides, games, and lights. Similarly, we were told we couldn't befriend kids from the local council estate, but of course, we did. And hanging around town on Saturdays? That was another no-go, but it didn't stop us from doing it whenever we could. Woolworths became a regular stop for us, where my friends and I would often engage in a bit of low-level shoplifting—something I'm not exactly proud of but was all part of our wild little lives at the time.

By today's standards, we were a bit feral, living out our private adventures in the absence of adult supervision. We did things that even by today's standards might raise eyebrows - like smoking by the time I was 10 years old. It's shocking to think back on it, but at the time, it was just another thing we did, a part of the rebellious freedom we enjoyed. Thankfully, I finally kicked that habit much later in life when COVID-19 hit, and I realized just how important my health was. But despite or because of all my early experiences those early years of pushing boundaries, getting into mischief, and carving out our own world of adventures are some of my fondest memories.

*[**Key Takeaway:** The foundations of health are laid early in life, but our ability to influence our well-being continues throughout our journey. My story demonstrates that while we may inherit certain predispositions, our lifestyle choices and responses to challenges play a crucial role in determining our health outcomes.]*

MS & ME

This perspective on my early years sets the stage for understanding not just how MS entered my life, but how my early experiences prepared me to face and manage this condition with resilience and determination.

MS & ME

Chapter 2

Down South

This particular chapter of my life was coming to an inevitable close. My parent's initial dream of emigrating to Australia had been abandoned, and instead, we found ourselves relocating to the heart of Somerset in South West England. For me, the move was nothing short of a massive culture shock, one that would shake the foundations of my young life. My mum had secured a teaching position at a small village primary school, and with that came another schoolhouse—yes, another one! My sister went off to art college in the nearest big town, my brother went to Liverpool to train with the Merchant Navy, and my father stayed behind in Scotland for another six months before finally joining us. Poor Nana, always the steadfast presence in our lives, also made the move with us, continuing to be a source of comfort, though she, too, must have felt the weight of this uprooting.

Living in that schoolhouse was an adjustment in itself, and not just because of the move to a new region. The house, though charming in its own right, came with an unusual set of challenges. The most notorious being the enormous spiders that seemed to invade our lives daily, crawling in from the graveyard next door. We four females—my mum, my sister, Nana, and I—lived in a constant state of fear, battling against these eight-legged intruders who seemed determined to terrorize us. The combination of living next to a graveyard and being overrun by spiders certainly added to the overall sense of discomfort in those early days of settling in.

[Health Context: Dr. Sarah Montgomery, a specialist in adolescent health, notes that major transitions during teenage years can create

prolonged stress responses that may influence autoimmune conditions later in life.]

For me, the hardest part of this move was not just the physical displacement but the emotional upheaval of leaving behind everything that was familiar and dear to me. My Scottish accent, once simply part of who I was, quickly became a source of ridicule and teasing from the local children. Somerset might have only been a few hundred miles away from Scotland, but it felt like a different world entirely. I had to take a bus to school every morning, a short three-mile journey that felt like a trek into a hostile environment where I stood out like a sore thumb. The local middle school had already established its friendship circles, and I was the outsider—the new kid with the strange accent. Finding my place was a daily struggle.

[Expert Insight: "Adolescent stress can fundamentally alter immune system function," notes Dr. Rebecca Chen, immunologist. "The teenage years represent a critical period when the body's stress response systems are still developing."]

The loneliness of that time hit me hard. I had left behind a circle of fabulous friends, especially my best friend, who had been my rock since early childhood and whose home had been another sanctuary. Now I found myself in a middle school where everyone else had already spent a year forging friendships, making it nearly impossible to break into any group. My accent didn't help matters, either. I became hyper-aware of the way I spoke, feeling self-conscious about every word that came out of my mouth. The isolation was palpable, and my only solace came from an unexpected friendship with a girl who lived at the Traveller's site on the edge of the village. Perhaps it was our shared sense of not belonging that drew us together, but she became my one companion during those difficult months. The other relationship that continued to give me so much comfort, was with my dog, Carly. We became inseparable discovering new places to explore together.

Meanwhile, my mother was going through her own transformation. She decided to pursue a conversion course that would allow her to teach at the secondary level in her true passion: Drama. It was a dream long deferred, as she had originally gone to Drama and Dance school in her teenage years, and now she was finally getting the opportunity to teach the subject she loved most. For her, this was a dream come true, but for the rest of us, it meant another upheaval.

With my mother's career shift came another move, this time to a village closer to the town where my sister was studying art. Once again, we packed up our lives and relocated, and once again, I was thrust into the challenge of starting over. This time, I joined a secondary school, but the situation was all too familiar. The students had already formed their tight-knit friendship groups, and I was left to navigate the tricky waters of fitting in as the "new girl" once again—this time with the added stigma of being the Scottish outsider.

The adjustment to secondary school was no easier than middle school had been. I was still the odd one out, the little alien girl with the unfamiliar accent, trying to find a place where I belonged. Every school I entered seemed to already have its established hierarchies and social structures, and I always seemed to be arriving too late to the party. The challenge of fitting in weighed heavily on me, and it was hard not to feel like an outsider looking in, especially when the kids in these schools had grown up together and already had their solid circles of friends.

Another contributing factor to my initial isolation during this time was my parents' rather misguided sense of snobbery, which, in retrospect, seemed both perplexing and unnecessary. For reasons I never fully understood, they were adamant that I should not attend the local secondary school where the other children from our village went. Instead, they insisted on enrolling me in a school five miles away, which only compounded the difficulties I was already facing. It was as if, in their attempt to give me what they thought was a "better" education or a more "refined" environment, they unintentionally made things harder for me.

By placing me in a school that none of the local children attended, I was essentially isolated on two fronts. Not only did I have to navigate the complex social landscape of a new school where I knew no one and where friendships had already been solidified long before I arrived, but I also had the added challenge of trying to fit in with the children in our new village. These were the kids I lived alongside, but I didn't go to school with them, so I existed in this strange in-between world, neither fully integrated into the social life of my school nor into the community life of my village.

The daily bus ride to school became a journey not just of miles but of emotional distance, as I felt increasingly disconnected from both worlds. At school, I struggled to break into established friendship circles. The children there already had shared histories, inside jokes, and a familiarity with one another that I simply didn't have. I was the outsider, the new girl, and on top of that, I had a thick Scottish accent that set me apart even further. No matter how hard I tried to blend in, I always felt like I was on the outskirts, watching friendships unfold from a distance.

At the same time, I faced the equally daunting challenge of trying to connect with the children in my home village. Since I wasn't attending school with them, I missed out on the shared experiences that typically bond kids together—those mundane yet significant moments like lunchtime chatter, after-school activities, or even the camaraderie of walking to and from school together. It was as if my life was split between two separate worlds, and I didn't fully belong in either of them.

While the children in my village were friendly enough, I always felt like a bit of an outsider in their midst, unable to fully immerse myself in their social dynamics because I wasn't part of their daily school life. They had their own tight-knit friendships, formed through the natural rhythm of seeing each other every day, and I was left trying to insert myself into their already-established social structure without the benefit of that shared routine.

These two moves in quick succession were a lonely and disorienting experience, to say the least. While most children my age were forging strong bonds through shared experiences, I was left navigating these fragmented social terrains, trying to carve out a place for myself where none seemed readily available. I often wondered why my parents had chosen this path for me, and though they likely believed they were doing what was best, their decision inadvertently heightened my sense of isolation. But even amid that struggle, I began to develop a resilience and inner strength that would serve me well in the years to come. Learning to adapt to new environments, no matter how difficult, became a skill I would carry with me for the rest of my life.

Thankfully, after a few uncomfortable years by the time I reached the age of fourteen, I finally felt as though I had found my place socially. I had strong friendship groups both at home and at school, and I no longer felt like the outsider I had once been. At home, the local Youth Club became the hub of our social lives. It was an eclectic group, with kids ranging from my age up to around twenty, which created a vibrant and dynamic mix of personalities, ages, and genders. There was always something happening, and being part of this lively group really seemed to suit my rebellious nature. Life felt exciting, full of possibility, and I had finally settled into a rhythm that felt right.

[Health Reflection: Looking back, I can identify several potential warning signs: frequent headaches, unexplained fatigue, and occasional muscle aches. While these symptoms seemed normal for a stressed teenager, they might have indicated early immune system dysregulation.]

[Medical Context: "Adolescent lifestyle choices, including sleep patterns and exposure to environmental toxins, can have lasting effects on immune system function," noted Dr. Sarah Peterson, a specialist in teenage health. "The body is particularly vulnerable to these influences during developmental years."]

By the time I turned sixteen, I had a moped of my own, which felt like a rite of passage into a new level of freedom and independence. Nearly all of us had motorbikes or mopeds and we would zip around from place to place, relishing the sense of freedom that those two wheels gave us. Our antics were typical of teenagers our age—getting into harmless trouble, experimenting with alcohol, and smoking whatever we could get our hands on. There were the occasional fights with kids from other villages, moments of bravado that now seem like part of the natural growing pains of adolescence. In many ways, we were just doing what most teenagers do: testing limits, exploring who we were, and having a bit of fun along the way.

School life was just as enjoyable, I had a solid circle of friends, and socially, things were finally falling into place. I even dated the most sought-after boy in school, the one everyone seemed to have their eye on, only to end the relationship on my own terms. It was one of those little teenage victories that felt monumental at the time, boosting my confidence and solidifying my place in the social hierarchy. My school friends and my village friends blended seamlessly, and for a while, life felt like it was on an upward trajectory. It was a good time, a moment of balance and belonging that had been missing in my earlier years of feeling out of place.

And then there was Carly, my ever-loyal Border Collie, who remained a constant source of comfort and companionship through it all. No matter what trouble I got into, Carly was always by my side. In fact, my parents knew me so well that whenever I was due for a stern lecture or "a good talking-to" about some misbehavior they'd caught wind of, Carly would be the first to suffer. My dad had a rule: if I was to be reprimanded, Carly had to be shut outside the house first, as if her presence would soften the blow of their scolding. She was my protector, my confidante, and my best friend, even if it meant she had to sit outside during my brushes with discipline.

Looking back on those years, they were formative in every sense. My rebellious streak had room to breathe within the safety of a supportive community, and while we may have been a bit wild, we were also just kids figuring out who we were. The mix of adventure, a bit of harmless trouble, and the sense of belonging to both a school and a village group gave me a newfound confidence and joy that I had not experienced since leaving my hometown in Scotland. It was a time of life when everything felt within reach, where friendships were strong, and where the world seemed wide open with possibilities.

(Health Context: Feeling a sense of belonging as a teenager is the foundation for building confidence and resilience. When teens find a community that accepts and values them, they not only discover who they are but also realize the strength that comes from authentic connections." Dr Lisa Damour, Adolescent Psychologist and Author)

MS & ME

At just sixteen and a half, I found myself moving yet again, but this time the circumstances were entirely different. I left behind the rural village life and relocated to a council house in the nearby town to live with my sister and her newborn child. It was a significant shift in more ways than one. My sister's pregnancy had been a source of immense tension within our family. Our parents, believing the situation was too difficult to manage, had tried to convince her to give the baby up for adoption. The pregnancy had progressed too far for an abortion, and this left my sister in emotional turmoil. Many sleepless nights were spent in our shared bedroom back in the village, as she wept and wrestled with the uncertainty of her future. I would lie awake, listening to her sob herself to sleep, feeling utterly helpless but determined to support her however I could.

When my sister decided to keep the baby, our lives took a dramatic turn. Moving in with her to help care for the child marked the beginning of a whole new chapter for me. It was an escape from the rigid rules of my parent's home and the start of a newfound freedom. Living with my sister meant I no longer had to navigate the expectations of my parents, instead, I was entering a world where I could begin to make my own decisions and explore what independence really felt like. The sense of liberation was exhilarating, despite the challenges that came with it.

But as with all transitions, it wasn't long before life shifted once again. My sister's boyfriend moved in, and I felt it was time for me to find a place of my own. I soon moved out and into a shared house, marking the start of what would become a period of financial hardship. Juggling multiple jobs became a necessity. I worked at a pub, despite being underage, pulling pints and serving locals well before I turned eighteen. On top of that, I found work at the local bingo hall and somehow managed to maintain a permanent job as well. It was a precarious balancing act, trying to make ends meet, and money was tight more often than not.

MS & ME

Dr. Julia Martin, an immunologist specializing in autoimmune disorders, explains: "During young adulthood, the body is still adapting to the hormonal and developmental changes of adolescence. Adding prolonged stress, erratic schedules, and environmental exposures can disrupt the body's natural immune regulation."

Despite my efforts, there were times when my financial situation became so dire that I had no choice but to return home to my parents, tail between my legs. By this point, they had relocated once again, this time to Devon, where they were busy developing a new home. Returning to them felt like a step backward, but it was a necessity when I found myself broke and unable to sustain the independence I had so eagerly sought. Their new life in Devon was different from the one we had known before, and while they were focused on their new project, I couldn't help but feel like I was treading water, trying to figure out how to stand on my own two feet.

This period of my life was marked by both a sense of freedom and the harsh realities of growing up. The move with my sister offered a taste of independence, but it also exposed me to the challenges of financial instability and the pressures of early adulthood. Working multiple jobs while trying to carve out my own path was exhausting, and the constant worry about money weighed heavily on me. Yet, in those difficult moments, I learned valuable lessons about resilience, resourcefulness, and the importance of perseverance. I had tasted freedom, but I had also come to understand the responsibilities that came with it. Each experience, from helping my sister through her pregnancy to managing on my own, shaped me in ways that would stay with me for the rest of my life.

In those final years, I spent in Somerset, my life became increasingly centered around the pub where I worked. It was more than just a job; it was a vibrant, exhilarating environment that felt alive with energy.

I quickly grew to love my role behind the bar, where I was not just serving drinks but becoming a part of the ever-changing backdrop of the pub's social scene. The pub had a certain rawness to it, an edge that made every shift feel like an adventure. I think my earlier years in the village, where I learned to hold my own and navigate complex social dynamics, prepared me for this new chapter. Those years taught me how to stand my ground and handle a wide array of personalities, which served me well in the often chaotic and unpredictable world of pub life.

Many of the kids I had grown up with in the village found their way to this same pub, continuing the bonds we had formed earlier in life. A lot of them were bikers, and this pub became their new hangout, the next stop in their journey toward adulthood. It wasn't just our small group, though; the pub attracted serious bikers from all over, and on weekends, it wasn't uncommon for Hell's Angels chapters from further east to roll in, their presence adding an extra layer of excitement and unpredictability to the atmosphere. The combination of live music, blaring jukeboxes, and the roar of motorbikes created an almost electric environment. It was loud, it was intense, and it felt like anything could happen at any moment.

Fights would occasionally break out, sometimes over petty squabbles and other times over more serious matters. The police were no strangers to the place, often making appearances when things got a little too wild. There were also plenty of drugs circulating, another element that added to the pub's rebellious edge. The air was thick with the sense that we were living on the fringe of society, part of a subculture that thrived on defiance and adrenaline. It was thrilling in a way that only youth can make it, and whilst I did like to dabble in drugs, I didn't get involved in anything too extreme. I was undeniably drawn to the excitement and freedom that came with being part of that world.

Around this time, my close friend moved to Bristol, and I started spending my weekends there. Bristol was a whole new scene. A larger, more cosmopolitan city with its own vibe. Compared to the small, insular life I had known in Somerset, Bristol felt like a breath of fresh air, an opportunity to expand my horizons. The more time I spent there, the more I realized that my hometown had given me all it could. I had grown restless, craving something bigger, something more than the familiar faces and routines that had shaped my life so far. Bristol represented a chance to reinvent myself, to break free from the past, and to step into a new chapter of my life.

And so, aged 20, in July of 1983, with that growing sense of anticipation, I decided to move to Bristol. It wasn't just a geographical move; it was symbolic of a larger shift in my life. Somerset had been a place of growth and learning, where I found my footing and discovered who I was. But now, I was ready for something more. Bristol offered the promise of new experiences, new people, and a world of possibilities that I was eager to explore. It was the beginning of an exciting new journey, and I couldn't wait to see where it would take me.

(Expert Insight: "The chaotic teenage years are like a storm that shapes the strongest trees. Navigating the turbulence of adolescence teaches flexibility, resilience, and the ability to adapt—essential skills that prepare teens to face and overcome life's challenges with confidence." – Dr. Gabor Maté, Physician and Trauma Expert.)

Chapter 3

City Life

If I remember correctly, I moved in June 1983. Here began a couple of years of nightclubs, again working in a pub, again holding down various full-time jobs, enjoying everything a big city has to offer. I loved the vibe of Bristol but I only had a few crazy months of single life before I met my life partner around November 1984, around forty years ago now! I had always probably drunk far too much in my teens but in Bristol, again working at a pub, it did define my life. Now I rarely drink. I remember going to the doctor as I had such bad stomach pains, beyond my usual horrendous period pains, only to be told that If I did not curb my lifestyle somewhat, I was heading for stomach ulcers! Really! age 20!

My friend and I shared a flat in the city, and one night, something extraordinary and inexplicable happened—something that I still struggle to fully comprehend to this day. It was an ordinary evening until we heard a loud noise, almost as if it were right at our back door. Startled, we rushed to investigate, expecting to find something mundane, but what we saw was anything but. Hovering above us was a large craft, it's surface alive with colourful lights whirring and spinning in a strange, rhythmic dance. I remember both of us standing there in stunned silence, completely transfixed, staring up at this craft with a mix of awe and confusion. The lights above us seemed otherworldly, casting strange shadows and colours across the night sky. We didn't speak, we didn't run—there was nothing but the two of us, frozen in place, gazing at this bizarre spectacle.

What's even stranger than the sight itself is what happened afterward—or rather, what didn't happen. Neither of us ever mentioned it again. Not that night, not the next day, not ever (almost!). We simply moved on as though nothing out of the ordinary had occurred, as though the experience had been erased from our conscious minds. I've thought about this encounter many times over the years, and it still puzzles me. Why didn't we talk about it? Was it too strange to process, or did we somehow convince ourselves it hadn't happened at all? Even as the years passed, the memory of that night remained vivid in my mind, though it sat in silence, unexplored, until much later in life.

I've always had a fascination with the supernatural, the occult, and the possibility of something beyond us humans. This incident only deepened that curiosity, though for a long time it remained a mysterious fragment of my past. It wasn't until several years later, after the birth of my son, that things took a darker turn. I began to suffer from horrendous night terrors, episodes so vivid and terrifying that they left me shaken for hours after waking. In these dreams, or perhaps hallucinations, I would find myself pinned to the bed, utterly unable to move or scream for help. It was as though an unseen force had total control over my body, trapping me in a state of paralysis. What was even more unsettling were the strobes of light that seemed to enter and exit my body during these episodes. The sensations were so intense, so real, that it was difficult to dismiss them as mere dreams.

[Medical Context: Night terrors and sleep paralysis, while not directly linked to MS, can be exacerbated by stress and fatigue—two factors often intertwined with autoimmune conditions.]

Over the years, I shared these experiences with my family, though they often responded with humour rather than concern. My kids, in particular, found it amusing, teasing me with jokes about alien abductions. "Oh, Mum thinks she was abducted by aliens!" they say with a laugh. And while I can see the humour in their reactions, for me, the experiences were definitely experienced at some level. I couldn't help but wonder if there was some connection between that strange encounter with the craft and the night terrors that followed years later. Had something happened that night that set these events in motion, or was it all just a figment of my imagination?

The mystery deepened even further around twenty years after that fateful encounter, during an unexpected visit from my old flatmate, who had, long since, moved away from Bristol. We were sitting around, chatting casually with my kids and husband, reminiscing about old times, and having a laugh about the C-3PO incident – see below!Out of nowhere, she brought up something that nearly stopped me in my tracks. "I think it was just a dream," she began, "but when we shared the flat, I remember us being disturbed by a loud noise at the back of the house. We went outside to check, and there was this flying saucer hovering over the roof!" My heart skipped a beat—her words mirrored the exact memory I had carried with me for all these years.

It was a moment of validation, a confirmation that I hadn't imagined the entire thing. For two decades, I had wondered whether that night had been real or just a strange dream, and here was my friend, unprompted, recalling the same event. She hadn't experienced the night terrors that plagued me in the years that followed, but her recollection of that night was enough to give credence to my own memories. What had we seen? Was it truly a flying saucer, or was it some strange shared hallucination? I still don't know the answer, but her words reignited the questions I had long pushed to the back of my mind.

Whether my experiences were real or simply products of my subconscious, that night left an indelible mark on me. I may never know if the craft we saw was of this world or another, and I may never fully understand the night terrors that haunted me after my son's birth. But one thing is certain: those experiences, strange as they were, remain a part of my story, a thread woven into the tapestry of my life that I will continue to unravel, piece by piece.

One of the funniest stories my husband loves to recount, without fail, in fact it's become something of a legend in our household, and it never fails to get a laugh. It all started the very first time he and his mate came over to our flat. My friend, who had a slim build, and I decided to have a little fun at their expense. I had recently bought a C-3PO costume as a gift for my nephew, who was absolutely obsessed with *Star Wars*. The idea of that golden droid must have sparked something mischievous in me because, after a few drinks and in high spirits, I convinced my friend to squeeze herself into the child-sized costume.

The sight was absolutely ridiculous - a young woman crammed into a C-3PO outfit designed for a child. My friend, always up for a laugh, played along perfectly, and we decided to surprise our guests. When the two young men walked into the room and saw this bizarre scene unfold before them, their faces were priceless. Their eyes widened in disbelief as they tried to make sense of what they were seeing—a *Star Wars* character brought to life in the most unexpected and silliest way possible.

To make matters even more absurd, we played it completely straight, as though there was nothing strange about the situation. The two men stood there, clearly bewildered, as my friend moved around in the golden suit, her limbs stiff like a robot, while I tried to keep a straight face. They didn't quite know how to react. And, unsurprisingly, they didn't stick around for very long! They left rather quickly, probably convinced that we were a couple of eccentric weirdos. Meanwhile, my friend and I were left in fits of laughter, absolutely cracking up over the whole thing.

MS & ME

For us, it was the height of hilarity—a ridiculous, spontaneous moment that became the foundation of a long-standing joke. But for my husband and his friend, it was undoubtedly a strange encounter. To this day, my husband still brings it up, shaking his head with a smile as he recalls how, at that moment, he was pretty certain we were completely mad. Yet, it didn't scare him off—if anything, it probably sealed the deal, as he got a glimpse of the fun and silliness that would become a staple of our relationship.

Looking back over the first two decades of my life, it's almost astonishing to realize that, despite the indulgence in alcohol and a fair share of unhealthy late-night snacks—kebabs at 4 a.m. come to mind—I managed to remain in relatively good health. It's not lost on me how fortunate I was, considering my lifestyle during those years wasn't exactly the epitome of wellness. The endless alcohol-fuelled nights out, cigarettes, and the poor food choices that followed could have easily taken a toll on my body. Yet, apart from a few minor ailments, I somehow sailed through that period with little to complain about health-wise. In retrospect, it almost feels like I dodged a bullet, given the reckless abandon with which I approached my health.

Overall, I consider myself incredibly lucky that, aside from terrible periods my health remained fairly resilient. Even as I think back to those carefree, and often careless, years of youth, it's almost surprising how well my body managed to keep up with me. Looking back now, I can't help but marvel at the balance between youthful invincibility and the grace of good fortune that seemed to carry me through. Even my lungs, which had already faced significant challenges at the beginning of my life, managed to hold their own despite the abuse I subjected them to through years of smoking. It's almost remarkable, considering how fragile they had once been, that they withstood the constant onslaught of cigarettes. It's a testament, perhaps, to the strength we sometimes take for granted in our bodies, even when we knowingly push them to their limits.

However, in hindsight, which is indeed, a wonderful thing, as my "health" luck was about to change.

Chapter 4

A Period of Settling

In April of 1986, after spending a couple of years hopping between various rented accommodations, Simon and I, finally took the plunge and bought our first home in the inner-city suburbs of Bristol. A step into a new chapter of our lives together, where we were putting down roots and carving out a space of our own on a Victorian terrace. The deposit was a gift from my nana and although she never traveled to visit our house, I am grateful she lived long enough to meet Dan, our firstborn child. This represented stability and the beginning of a new adventure in homeownership. We were excited to make it our own and had high hopes for this new chapter. At this point, I simply cannot ignore the undeniable fact: our eldest son is the living, breathing mirror image of his father, who is most definitely of this world!

However, our time in that house was cut short by a disturbing and unsettling situation. A year after settling into our new home, we made the difficult decision to move again, this time to the northern suburbs of the city. The reason? For several months, I found myself the target of a stalker, an experience that filled my mornings with dread. Every day, Simon would leave for work around 6 a.m., and I would take our rescue terrier out for a walk, thinking it would be a peaceful start to my day. But most mornings were anything but peaceful. I soon noticed that I was being followed by a kerb crawler, a man who seemed to appear almost out of nowhere, tailing me as I walked the dog.

At first, I tried to ignore him, hoping that it was just a one-off incident, but it soon became clear that he was having far too much fun. Almost every morning, he would trail behind me, shouting lewd and sexual insults in my direction, making what should have been a simple walk with the dog a nerve-wracking ordeal. His presence became a constant source of fear and anxiety, and I dreaded leaving the house in the mornings. I attempted to seek help from the authorities, desperately hoping for some kind of intervention or support from the police. But, to my dismay, my pleas for assistance were met with indifference. Despite the seriousness of the situation, there was little to no action taken to address the harassment I was enduring. With no help in sight and the situation growing increasingly unbearable, Simon and I realized that our only option was to move. We couldn't continue to live in an environment where I felt unsafe in my own neighbourhood. so, we packed up and relocated to the northern suburbs.

No sooner had we settled into our new home when it became clear that life had another unexpected twist in store for us—I was pregnant. It wasn't something we had planned, especially not so soon after committing to a bigger mortgage and the financial responsibilities that came with it. The news was both a surprise and a source of mixed emotions. We were excited, of course, but the timing felt overwhelming. Nevertheless, we quickly adjusted to the idea, and I set about preparing for the arrival of our child while continuing to work full-time.

Throughout the pregnancy, I remained committed to my job, working right up until the final days before our son was born. There was no extended maternity leave for me—just the minimum time off that I could afford before I had to return to work. I had to juggle the realities of impending motherhood with the pressures of my office job, and it felt like a constant balancing act.

[Medical Perspective: Current research shows that pregnancy can have a temporary protective effect on MS symptoms due to hormonal

changes, particularly in the third trimester. However, the postpartum period often brings a heightened risk of relapse.]

The birth itself was nothing short of dramatic, like a scene straight out of an episode of *E/R, the Chicago-based sitcom!*

After hours of labour with little to no progression, I found myself strapped to a monitor, confined to the bed, and unable to move. The medical staff were concerned about my lack of progress, and the more time passed, the more the situation escalated. An epidural was administered, but rather than providing relief, it seemed to complicate matters. Both my heart rate and the baby's began to show signs of distress, and suddenly, what had started as a hopeful labour turned into a terrifying ordeal.

I remember the moment vividly: the frantic urgency in the room, the anxious looks exchanged between the doctors and nurses as the heart rates dropped. The decision was made to rush me through those double doors to the operating theatre for an emergency C-section. The speed at which everything happened was overwhelming—one moment I was lying there, waiting and hoping for things to progress naturally, and the next, I was being rushed into surgery. It all felt like a blur, a whirlwind of activity as they prepared for the procedure, and before I knew it, my son was delivered safely into the world.

The experience, while harrowing, ended in relief. Despite the fear and uncertainty that surrounded the birth, both my son and I made it through safely. But the memory of that day remains vivid, etched into my mind as one of the most intense moments of my life—a mixture of joy, fear, and exhaustion, all wrapped into one unforgettable experience. Poor little Dan was absolutely covered in excrement, with it finding its way into every fold and crevice of his long, tiny body. It felt like it took days of careful washing to finally get him clean! Despite that messy beginning, he was a healthy and strong baby, full of life and resilience from the very start.

Those years spent working in an endlessly monotonous office job, with only the weekends to look forward to, were a wake-up call for me. The predictability of the routine and the lack of fulfilment made me realize that I was meant for something more, something with purpose and meaning. I had wasted my teenage years at college, more interested in earning money and spending time at the pub than actually focusing on my studies. At the time, I was young and carefree, and the excitement of those years had seemed like enough. But as time went on, I found myself yearning for more than just fleeting moments of fun—I wanted a real career, something I could be proud of.

Determined to change the course of my life, I decided to go back to college. I set my sights on gaining qualifications that would open doors to a more fulfilling future. With Dan still a little one, I managed to balance my responsibilities as a mother by attending college one day a week and bringing him with me to the crèche. It wasn't easy, but it felt like I was finally moving in the right direction. Over the next two years, I worked hard and earned a BTec in Business Studies with distinction. It was a moment of pride, a sign that I could achieve something meaningful, and it gave me the confidence to aim higher.

By 1992, with Daniel nearly five years old, I decided to take the next step and apply to university to pursue a teaching degree. I enrolled in a B.Ed. Hons program in Business Education, eager to turn my academic achievements into a career. In all honesty, my heart had always leaned toward something more creative. I would have preferred to pursue a teaching qualification in a more artistic or imaginative field, but my qualifications were in business, and that was the path available to me at the time for secondary teaching. So,

I embraced it, knowing that this was the opportunity I had, and determined to make the most of it.

I finally felt like I was on a path that aligned with my desire for a career. It wasn't the creative outlet I had envisioned, but it was a start, and it allowed me to balance my roles as both a mother and a student, slowly building the foundation for the future I truly wanted.

About a year into my time at university, something rather impulsive—and, in hindsight, perhaps a bit reckless—stirred within me. I had settled into the rhythm of my studies and found the academic demands manageable. Amid it all, I started to feel like everything was going smoothly, almost too smoothly. Somewhere deep down, I convinced us both that we could handle more, and that maybe, just maybe, it was the right time for Dan to have a sibling. It seemed like a perfectly reasonable idea at the time, even though I was still in the middle of my degree. So, with that thought in mind, baby number two was conceived almost on cue, arriving right on schedule at the end of my first year's summer holiday, in September of 1993.

This time, much like the first, the delivery wasn't straightforward. Once again, I found myself undergoing an emergency C-section, a repeat of the frantic rush and medical intervention that had marked Dan's birth. Even though I had been through it before, it was still a challenging experience, both physically and emotionally. However, by this point, I had become somewhat accustomed to juggling the demands of life, motherhood, and my education. I knew it wasn't going to be easy balancing a new baby, a young child, and university, but I felt a strange sense of determination, convinced that I could manage it all. Of course, the reality was as demanding as I had anticipated, but I wasn't alone in facing those challenges. Thankfully, their father was an equal partner then and ever since, when it came to parenting, sharing responsibilities made an enormous difference, if I were to compare us to other couples. He was hands-on and supportive, which lightened the load considerably. But beyond his help, I was fortunate enough to have a couple of incredibly reliable friends who stepped up during those difficult years. One was a university mate, someone who understood the unique pressures of balancing motherhood with academic life, and the other was an old friend from my old workplace.

With none of my family living nearby, these friends became my lifeline. Their support was invaluable, whether it was helping with the kids, offering a sympathetic ear, or simply providing a much-needed break when things got overwhelming. I quickly realized that I couldn't have managed without them, and their kindness and generosity were crucial in allowing me to continue pursuing my degree while raising three young children (one is still to arrive!). Looking back, I'm deeply grateful for their friendship and the way they rallied around me when I needed it most.

Chapter 5

The Diagnosis

From the beginning of my third year at University, I had also been working as a lecturer at the college where I had completed my studies. Money was always so tight. Simon had been made redundant the year Joss was born and had to take a much lower-paid job. So here we were juggling Uni lectures, teaching hours, childcare and Simon's new job that was shift work and worse still, often nights. We were living in a house that was in negative equity and living from pay cheques to pay cheques. It was hard it was darn right horrible. When you are in that perpetual struggle sometimes you are just on autopilot, seeing nothing other than getting through the day.

(Medical Insight: "Financial stress is one of the most significant factors affecting overall health. Chronic worry about money can lead to elevated cortisol levels, disrupting sleep, increasing blood pressure, and contributing to anxiety, depression, and even cardiovascular disease. Addressing financial challenges holistically is essential for maintaining both mental and physical well-being." – Dr. Robert Sapolsky, Neuroscientist and Stress Expert)

I distinctly remember driving home from teaching night class and just wanting to keep driving, tears flowing down my cheeks, but numb of all feelings. This weird feeling of having not an ounce of energy to feel anything other than getting through the day, to get to the next day. I don't think I had ever before or since felt that low. The end of the Uni-term arrived and then a few weeks later my contracted teaching hours ended – relax. Then it all became apparent – yep! You guessed it, baby number three was on her way.

MS & ME

She arrived just at the beginning of the four weeks of the Christmas holiday, this time a planned C Section. Taken from my womb and placed into my arms, our daughter had arrived. I could have chosen the 6th of the month for this event, but as both the boys had arrived of their own accord on the 7th, the 7th it was. In January 1996, my final year of university, just as I had done before, here I was breastfeeding at the back of the lecture hall.

I thought this tumultuous period was nearly over, the finale getting ever closer. There were just a few short months to go, and all the sacrifices would be worth it! Then a new problem became apparent creeping up and biting me on the bum, just as I was thinking the worst was over. Now I found myself struggling through with a dodgy right arm, devoid of normal feeling. The other girls in my cohort were such a great support. Until then I had been the mummy of our small female student group, being the eldest aged 33, but now the tables turned in my favour and they really helped me. Holding the baby was harrowing enough in my right arm, but holding a pen was just the weirdest sensation! Lecture notes were shared with me and luckily my final dissertation was already underway. I had not been able to complete my final teaching practice so that was playing on my mind, but I knew I just had to get through those last months to graduate with my peers!

I had to cancel my fourth-year teaching practice that had been organised in a secondary school. It was an eight-week experience that would have taken me beyond the baby's due date so had not been possible, I was now faced with the task of re-organizing this, a crucial step in completing my degree. I had completed a successful second year vocational in the Further Education college where I had completed my higher education just two years prior. Also, the same college where I had obtained paid work as a lecturer ever since that practice. Some of the mature male students in my cohort had followed a similar path and had returned to FE for their final practice so I saw no reason I could not do the same. However, things did not go as smoothly as I had hoped. To my frustration, in that last period at university when I had thought I was finally on the home straight, another lecturer, who had some influence over the decision-making process, was adamantly opposed to the idea of me completing my teaching practice in an FE college. His resistance felt unjustified and unreasonable, and as the situation escalated, it became an increasingly unpleasant experience. I was already struggling physically but I was determined not to back down. I had only just regained normal feeling in my right hand and arm and now I had a new fight on my hands. After hearing accounts of his derogatory references to my domestic situation, I decided to take the matter up with the University Dean, formally raising a case of discrimination. Unfortunately, the case didn't go in my favour, and the hierarchy ultimately sided with the opposing lecturer. It was a bitter pill to swallow. Thankfully, not all was lost. My personal tutor, who had supported me throughout the four years, stepped in and advocated on my behalf. His support proved to be invaluable. With his help, I was able to secure a placement at the FE college, allowing me to complete my practice hours in the environment where I felt most at home. Most of my hours were fulfilled in the mornings, and I continued teaching evening classes as well, balancing both in a way that worked for me and my family. What could have been a major setback turned into a victory, thanks to the support of my tutor and my own persistence.

Many long days ensued, whilst I grappled with finishing all my work for the university, preparing for my forthcoming, final teaching practice, and continuing the balancing act of childcare and family life with a newborn, a two-year-old, and an eight-year-old. I really could not believe how I managed to finish my honours degree at the same time as my fellow students with a 2.1 honours degree. I am rarely a spiteful person, but when I landed a top job at one of the best schools in my area it was certainly an "up yours" to the university lecturer who had put me through so much hell in those final months.

In September 1996, I started my career as a fully-fledged teacher. Two incomes at last, enough spare cash to look after our childcare requirements. It certainly was not easy, but it was a fulfilling time. I loved teaching, the contact with the pupils, building strong camaraderie with my fellow teachers, and planning exciting lessons and trips. But after being a parent it is a challenging and exhausting vocation. I fully immersed myself in school life, taking on extra responsibilities and working long hours. But these things took their toll, and it soon became apparent that this level of commitment was unsustainable.

The fact that my sister had already been diagnosed with MS in the early 90's just as I had been carving out my career meant that I knew what the signs and symptoms were. Each time I had one of my episodes, deep down I knew what was coming. I had mentioned my sister's diagnosis to my doctor on my visit regarding the sensory disturbance in my arm and hand. From recollection, I was told to go back if it didn't pass in a couple of weeks. MS is often diagnosed retrospectively, a process that can drag on as doctors wait for the right combination of symptoms to appear, or until they can finally coax you into the MRI machine for a definitive scan. In my case, it seems I had experienced subtle symptoms leading up to the more serious event that eventually revealed the full picture. There were signs I could have paid more attention to, but at the time, they seemed too minor to raise alarm. I recall several instances where certain areas of my body would inexplicably lose sensation—nothing that affected my mobility, but rather small, localized patches of numbness, particularly on my right leg. These numb spots felt strange and a bit concerning, but easy to ignore. I dismissed them, figuring they were one of those curious, fleeting bodily quirks that come and go.

[Medical Context: Relapsing-Remitting MS (RRMS) accounts for about 85% of initial MS diagnosis. Advances in diagnostic tools like MRI scans and spinal fluid tests have improved early detection, but the variability of symptoms makes it a challenging disease to diagnose and treat.]

However, what happened in the spring of 1999 was an entirely unique experience—one that couldn't be brushed aside. It was as if my body had been quietly whispering its warning signs for years, and suddenly it decided to scream. The first alarming symptom was double vision. I remember standing at my bedroom window, feeling unsteady and disoriented, and gazing out across the golf course toward the line of Poplar trees that formed the horizon. I blinked, confused and frightened, as I realized my vision was duplicating the trees before me. Seeing two of everything was terrifying, and I felt an overwhelming sense of panic creeping in. Every bodily function is important, and it's distressing when any of them malfunction, but there was something particularly horrifying about my vision failing. I could not trust what my eyes were showing me, and the disorientation that followed was unbearable. All I wanted to do was close my eyes and hide from it.

At the same time, my body began to betray me in other ways. A weakness crept into my right side, something I had never experienced before. That morning, even brushing my teeth became a monumental struggle. My arm felt heavy and uncooperative, and my whole body seemed to be enveloped in a fog of weakness and helplessness that I had never known. It was devastating—a loss of control over my own body that was as frightening as it was debilitating. I felt like I was collapsing inward, unable to muster the strength to function, let alone understand what was happening.

MS & ME

At that moment, I was completely dependent on my husband, Simon. The simple task of calling in sick to my school was too much for me to handle, so I had to ask him to do it for me. He also made an urgent call to our doctor, securing me an appointment. Thankfully, Simon was working the afternoon shift at the time, which meant he was home with me on that terrifying morning—he was there to witness the beginning of what would become a life-changing ordeal. I was fortunate to have his presence and support, but it was still a moment that fundamentally altered the course of our lives. The symptoms of that spring day were so vastly different from the minor numbness I had experienced before. This was a full-blown assault on my body, and from that day forward, nothing would be quite the same.

[Medical Context: MS is a chronic autoimmune disease where the immune system attacks the myelin sheath protecting nerve fibers. This leads to a wide range of symptoms, including fatigue, vision problems, and motor weakness. Treatment focuses on managing symptoms and slowing disease progression.]

That first major relapse I experienced lasted around three months from February to April. I've never allowed myself to dwell too much on that period, nor have I ever let it define me. In fact, I've made a conscious effort not to let it overshadow my life. The only reason I even remember the time of year is because I returned to my job at school immediately after the Easter school holidays. Thankfully, by the Easter holiday, I was well enough to have our planned family holiday to North Wales.

I took advantage of the services offered at the MS Centre, even before receiving a formal diagnosis, as I had been recommended to use the available facilities. The holistic treatments were exemplary, with the oxygen tank being one of the most prominent options. However, my claustrophobia meant this therapy caused me more stress than benefit. While other service users experienced great results, it simply wasn't for me.

What truly proved to be a great therapy for the whole family was seeing the advert for puppies at a farm that we passed on our journey to the MS Centre on our weekly visits. Our gorgeous Springer Spaniel puppy. Bringing so much joy to the whole family, the puppy encouraged daily walks, as we had been without a dog for a couple of years this was a welcomed exercise. Although taxing at times, these walks gave me the fresh air and nature fix that is so vital for overall well-being.

Returning to the normality of work was such a relief. The school's management team was incredibly supportive during this time, for which I am endlessly grateful. They created an environment where I felt comfortable taking rest days when necessary, without the overwhelming sense of guilt that usually accompanies time off for illness. It was such a relief to know that I wasn't being judged for prioritizing my health. Even so, I knew deep down that I couldn't continue in the same way forever. Teaching is, without a doubt, a vocation—something you pour your heart and soul into, giving your very best to your students. And though I loved the profession, I came to the difficult realization that I could no longer sustain that level of commitment.

The decision didn't come easily, but I knew I had to make a significant change for the sake of my health and well-being. I handed in my resignation immediately after Easter one year after that first relapse, in 2000. By the end of that summer term, my teaching career had come to a close. It was a bittersweet moment—letting go of something I was so enthusiastic about and had worked so hard to achieve. But also accepting the reality that I needed to focus on my health and adapt to the changes MS was bringing to my life. Though I left the classroom, I never let go of the lessons I learned through teaching, and it remains a cherished chapter in my life, even as I moved on to new horizons. To this day I have young men and women approach me to tell me how their lives are turning out and reminding me of our days together as teacher and pupil. It is such an honour to have played a small part in helping shape their lives and dreams, nothing is more fulfilling than making a positive and lasting effect on the life of another.

*[**Stress and MS**: Research shows that chronic stress can exacerbate MS symptoms by increasing inflammation and weakening the immune system. Managing stress through mindfulness, delegation, and clear boundaries is critical for long-term health.]*

Chapter 6

A woman's home is Her Mansion

Two other significant and exciting events unfolded in that new millennium marking the new chapter in my life. First, during the Easter holidays, we got married, solidifying a relationship that had already been such a solid foundation for our family. The second was the beginning of a new career path. Upon returning to school after the break, I handed in my resignation, as I was about to embark on an exciting venture as the Director of my own business. The transition to being self-employed wasn't without its challenges, though. There's no guidebook for becoming your own boss, and while autonomy is certainly a welcome change, it comes with its own unique stresses. Yet, this new phase of life brought a sense of freedom and control that I hadn't experienced before, and I embraced the opportunity.

This stage of my life, which lasted approximately eleven years, was defined by growth and change—both personally and professionally. Our children were growing up, filling our home with the laughter and energy that only children can bring. Our Springer Spaniel was always by our sides, and our cat, who is still with us to this day, added to the warmth of our home. Amidst the hustle and bustle of running a business and raising a family, I also had the good fortune of living in Bristol, which, as it turns out, was close to a world-renowned Multiple Sclerosis (MS) research department at the local hospital. In the early 2000s, I was fortunate to be selected for a trial of a disease-modifying drug. Looking back, I believe one of the reasons I was chosen was because I had a young family, and the doctors likely saw the importance of managing my symptoms as best as possible.

MS & ME

The treatment required daily injections, which I had to administer myself. It became a strict routine—I had to rotate the injection sites between my arms, thighs, stomach, and even my bum, repeating the cycle each week. Interestingly, this new regimen began right around the Easter holiday once again. I remember this so clearly because shortly after starting the injections, I experienced a sudden boost of energy. I had tried the Hyperbaric Oxygen tank in the late 90's whilst off school for those three months, as many people had claimed relief from the fatigue. But being claustrophobic, this particular therapy was not for me. Once again, a big positive did arise from our weekly trips to the MS Centre and that was our gorgeous Springer Spaniel pup, who grew up with our children and was a much-loved addition to our family.

Thankfully, the new injection regime made me for the first time in what felt like forever, have enough stamina for a proper family day out. We decided to take the kids to a theme park, but the day wasn't without its dramatic moments. One particular ride, the Pirate Ship, gave us an experience we'll never forget. It was one of those classic rides that swings back and forth, gaining momentum until you're nearly vertical. What started as fun quickly turned into sheer terror when Esme began to slip beneath the safety bar. In that heart-stopping moment, I realized just how important my newfound strength was. As gravity tried to pull her from my arms, I clung to her with all the strength I could muster, holding her securely against the force. She was screaming, tears streaming down her face, and all I could think about was keeping her safe until the ride mercifully ended. Those three minutes felt like an eternity, and by the time it was over, we were all shaken, but safe. We all disembarked in silence until we reached a nearby bench that represented sanctuary, at least it was static, where Simon and I were almost hysterical in our relief. We laugh about it now, but at the time, it was terrifying. The memory of that day is forever etched in my mind, a combination of pride in my physical strength and the fear of what could have happened on that terrifying ride.

During those years, I experienced a handful of minor MS relapses, but thankfully, none that were life-altering or completely debilitating. My focus during that period was firmly on building my business—a conference centre located on the outskirts of the city, which was steadily growing into a successful venture. In the early days, the workload was, frankly, overwhelming. The physical demands of setting up rooms for events, managing the logistics, and keeping everything clean were part and parcel of the daily grind. My business partner and I handled all of these tasks ourselves in those initial years. We had to wear multiple hats and dig deep to keep everything running smoothly.

However, as the business began to flourish, the pressure gradually lifted. We were finally able to hire staff, which allowed us to delegate some of the more physically demanding tasks. With a team in place, we could step back from the daily grind and focus on the bigger picture. Our attention shifted to the strategic aspects of the business—marketing, client relations, and ensuring that the company continued to grow in the right direction. It was a huge relief to step away from the exhausting manual work, but there was also a profound sense of pride that came with it. We had built something real and sustainable, a business that reflected all the hard work, sacrifice, and dedication we had invested. Watching it thrive was immensely rewarding.

Even with the progress I made in the business, MS never completely disappeared from my life. It had a way of making its presence known, reminding me that it was always lurking in the background. One particularly memorable episode involved a strange sensation in my face. I remember standing in front of the mirror, noticing that one side of my face was drooping as if I had suffered a stroke. My colleagues were far more alarmed than I was, rushing to express their concern. However, I remained calm, instinctively knowing that this was yet another symptom of my MS. It lasted for about a week, during which I continued to go to work each day, though I kept a low profile. I spent more time than usual tucked away in the office, not out of fear, but out of vanity. I wasn't too keen on anyone seeing me with half of my face sagging! Fortunately, the episode passed as quickly as it had appeared, and life soon returned to its usual rhythm.

*[**Medical Context**: Facial weakness or drooping, often mistaken for a stroke, can be a symptom of MS due to nerve inflammation. These episodes, while alarming, are typically temporary and improve as inflammation subsides.]*

Beyond that incident, most of my MS symptoms during those years were manageable, and fatigue was much reduced. I experienced what I referred to as "mushy feet syndrome," a strange, indescribable sensation that felt like I was walking on soggy moss and a hot oil feeling dripping from the base of my spine down the back of my legs. This would usually happen when I pushed myself too hard physically or overextended myself at work. Alongside that sensation was an uncomfortable feeling of being tightly wrapped in an invisible corset, particularly around my upper abdomen. These symptoms, while unsettling, became a part of my reality. I learned to adapt to them, treating them more as challenges to be managed rather than obstacles that would define or limit my life. During my years teaching I had had little time for socialising but now when I didn't have the burden of marking and lesson preparation, I could at least now make time to nurture friendships and we were able to enjoy a great social life with friends and neighbours whilst the kids played out in the close where we lived.

MS & ME

The years I spent running the conference centre were filled with joy, growth, and unforgettable memories. Managing the beautiful mansion house where the business was based gave me a deep sense of pride and ownership. I loved walking through the grounds with our family dog, soaking in the peaceful surroundings, or playing hide-and-seek with the kids in the grand, yet sometimes eerily spooky, old building. We hosted weddings, parties, and even my son's 18th birthday, which was a celebration to remember. My dad and I shared a joint party for my 40th birthday and his 70th, I was so proud to showcase my business to so many families and friends of mine and my parents. Running the conference centre brought me into contact with so many different people and their businesses, opening my eyes to the sheer variety of industries and professions out there. In fact, I often joke that I could write an entire book based on all the fascinating clients we worked with over the years.

One of the most memorable—and hilarious—moments came when my business partner excitedly told me that M&S, or Marks & Spencer, was coming for a viewing. We were thrilled at the thought of such a prestigious company wanting to use our venue! We even had a light-hearted argument about who would have the honour of showing them around. I reminded her of a time when we had both competed to show a handsome young client around, only for her to return with a "Hitler moustache" of coffee granules stuck to her sweaty upper lip after refilling a coffee pot. We laughed ourselves silly at the memory, and eventually, I won the debate. I would be the one to greet the esteemed M&S representatives.

But when the front door opened, I was in for a shock. It was immediately clear that these visitors were not from Marks & Spencer! Trying to keep a straight face was almost impossible. The man who entered was the tallest, slimmest person I had ever seen, wearing tiny round sunglasses and chains hanging from his jeans. The woman accompanying him wore a skirt so short it defied belief.

Conducting the tour without letting my amusement show was a true test of my professionalism. They seemed particularly interested in the size and access of our cellar rather than the beautifully appointed meeting rooms. It only took seconds to realize that these guests were not from M&S at all, but from S&M! Needless to say, much to the disappointment of our husbands, we had to decline their offer to book the cellar for their unusual event. It was one of those moments that seemed absurd at the time but has since become a favourite story to tell, always met with laughter.

Looking back, those years were marked by growth, challenges, and resilience. Running a business, raising a young family, and managing the ever-present realities of MS was no easy feat. But I came through it stronger, more determined, and with a clearer sense of what I was capable of. The journey was not always smooth, but it was uniquely mine. I navigated it with the support of Simon and our friends, a lot of grit, and a good dose of humour to carry me through the tough times.

When the global financial crash hit in 2008, the business took a significant blow. We were faced with some tough decisions regarding the mansion house. It quickly became clear that it was no longer financially viable for both my business partner and me to draw an income from the business. After much deliberation, I made the difficult decision to buy her out and continue running the business on my own, with a small, dedicated team. While it was daunting to take on the full responsibility, I relished the autonomy that came with running the venture solo. The following years were both rewarding and exhausting, but I loved being fully in control of the business's success.

Eventually, however, the time came for the mansion and me to part ways. In June 2011, I left the property for the last time, marking the end of a significant chapter in my life. For the three months since receiving notice from my landlords, I had desperately searched for a new venue to keep the business going, but nothing seemed to fit. It was with a heavy heart that I made one of my closest friends redundant and ultimately closed the business. Those eleven years had been some of the most rewarding and memorable of my life and saying goodbye to them was incredibly difficult. My days of being the "lady of the manor" had come to an end, and I mourned them deeply. However, the memories and lessons from that period remain with me always, shaping the person I am today. The fondness I feel for those 11 years in charge of my own mansion house, walking the grounds with our dog, playing hide and seek with the kids in the beautiful, yet sometimes spooky building, having parties for all our friends, holding wedding parties, my son's 18th party is always so much fun. Having a conference centre brings you in contact with so many people and their lives, it really opens your eyes to all the other businesses out there that use your services (in fact I could write a book just about that!)

(Expert Insight: "True business fulfillment comes when passion meets purpose, creating value not just for profit but for people. The joy of achievement lies in knowing your work makes a difference and inspires others to do the same." – Sir Richard Branson, Entrepreneur and Founder of Virgin Group)

MS & ME

Chapter 7

Anyone for coffee

So, a new business venture dawned, and with it came a sense of excitement and purpose. I've always thrived on being around people, and somewhere along the way, the idea formed in my mind that owning a small café in the heart of the community was the perfect next step. It seemed idyllic—a chance to create a warm, welcoming space where people could gather. So, I threw myself into building this new business, brimming with idealistic enthusiasm. But, oh, how naive I was! Little did I realize that running a café would turn out to be one of the hardest undertakings I'd ever attempted. In fact, getting that little shop unit ready for opening nearly cost as much as setting up my 11-room conference centre!

Every step of the way was a challenge. From negotiating with builders and plumbers to managing the three-month whirlwind timeline before the grand opening, it felt like I was carrying the weight of the world on my shoulders. There was no room for mistakes, as everything I owned and had earned from the success of my previous business was at risk. I endured sleepless nights, lying awake worrying about whether the tradesmen would meet their deadlines or if something would go catastrophically wrong at the last minute. In hindsight, I wonder what planet I was on when I thought this new endeavour would be a charming, easy-going venture! It was a gruelling process, but after what felt like a Herculean effort, we finally opened the café on January 7, 2012.

Lesson here, be careful what you wish for!

The night before opening was a blur—we didn't get to bed until 3 a.m., and by 8:30 that same morning, we were opening the doors to the public. To my astonishment, we had built so much interest in the community that there were literally queues outside, eager to see what we had created. It was a whirlwind of a day, full of chaos, excitement, and an incredible amount of support. My staff, who had stuck with me through all the delays and setbacks, were nothing short of amazing. We were exhausted by the end of it, but also exhilarated by the day's success. We even had record-breaking takings that day, and as we all went home, drained but happy, I felt a deep sense of accomplishment.

Amid all this, around the same time, my MS treatments took a new and challenging turn. My consultant changed my daily cutaneous injections to a new regimen: deep muscle injections once a week. These injections were far more painful, and they required Simon to administer them, as I couldn't bring myself to handle the thick needles. The injections alternated between the tops of my legs each week, and the pain was excruciating. To make matters worse, I would experience flu-like symptoms every time I had one. It became a weekly ordeal—preparing for the injections by taking anti-inflammatory tablets and paracetamol, knowing full well what was coming. Those deep muscle injections, along with the body scans I had to endure, were some of the worst experiences I've had with MS. But, despite the pain, I count myself lucky compared to the treatment's others have to face.

I spent seven years nurturing the business. And yes, seven is a significant number in my life—every one of my children was born on the 7th of the month, and this number seems to weave its way through my life with surprising regularity! There were so many aspects of the café that I truly loved. My staff were fantastic, and we always had a fresh stream of youngsters working Saturdays, as well as students from local schools completing their work experience placements. Just as I had done at the conference centre, I made sure we provided our own training. It was incredibly fulfilling to be at the heart of a small community, building real connections with people, and in many cases, being their only point of human contact from one day to the next.

Running the café gave me a deeper understanding of the hardships people face. Working in that space, I encountered people from all walks of life—some struggling with homelessness, others battling mental or physical health issues. Seeing their resilience taught me a lot about humility and compassion. It was a reminder that we often have no idea what burdens others are carrying. Through the café, I was able to be part of their lives, even in small ways, and that was something I cherished.

I also worked with two of my three children during this time, which was both a blessing and a challenge. On one hand, I was so grateful for their support, but on the other, I worried that working at the café might be holding them back from finding their own paths in the world. Nevertheless, we made it work. Simon would come in to help on Saturdays, and sometimes we would work together on Sundays, preparing and serving Sunday lunches. We were a good team, in the café as well as in life, and there was something incredibly satisfying about working side by side to keep the business running.

By the time we opened the café, I was older—49 to be exact. Time, as it does for all of us, had moved on, and though I felt ready for this new chapter, I soon realized that age had begun to take a greater toll on my body. I had always worked hard, and during my years running the conference centre, I often pushed myself to the very edge of what my body could handle. There were days when I would drive home in tears, utterly exhausted, both physically and mentally, from the demands of the day. But looking back, even those challenging times paled in comparison to what the café required of me.

If you can't stand the heat keep out of the kitchen:

MS & ME

(Expert Insight: "Excessive heat can significantly impact individuals with MS, as it often exacerbates symptoms like fatigue, weakness, and cognitive challenges. Keeping cool is not just about comfort—it's essential for maintaining function and overall well-being." – Dr. Nicholas LaRocca, Multiple Sclerosis Researcher and Advocate)

The toll the café took on me was unlike anything I had experienced before. The heat would consume my body, zapping my energy, my legs aching and weak with exhaustion. Crying became almost second nature, a default response to the overwhelming fatigue that consumed me. I would wake up in the morning already dreading the day ahead, tears welling up at the thought of facing yet another round of relentless challenges. As I stood at the cleaning station in the corner of the café, washing mountains of dishes, I would cry silently, hoping the steam from the sink would mask my tears. It became a routine: putting on a brave face for the customers, smiling through the pain, pretending that everything was fine. But beneath that façade, I was falling apart.

During this time, as if the emotional roller coaster of running the café wasn't enough, I faced another deeply personal and heart-wrenching challenge—my dad passed away after a two-year battle with Still's Disease. His illness had been a long and painful struggle, one that weighed heavily on the entire family. We watched as the once strong and vibrant man we knew was gradually worn down by this rare and relentless condition, an artist no longer able to hold a pencil or paintbrush. Despite our hopes for recovery, the disease eventually took his life.

The news of his diagnosis had shaken all of us, but we rallied together to support my parents in every way we could. The family became a source of strength, not just for my father, but for each other. We navigated the difficult terrain of hospital visits, doctors' appointments, and the ups and downs of his treatment. Still's Disease, with its unpredictable flare-ups, had moments of false hope when things seemed to improve, only to be followed by periods of rapid decline. Each new symptom felt like another blow, and while we held onto hope, there was an unspoken understanding that time was not on our side.

What made the situation even more poignant was the fact that my parents had only recently returned to the UK after spending 18 wonderful years living in France. They had loved their time there, embracing the peaceful, sun-drenched life that France offered. The move back to the UK had been intended as a new chapter in their lives, a chance to reconnect with family and settle into a slower pace as they grew older. But instead of the fresh start they had envisioned, they found themselves grappling with the harsh realities of my father's declining health. The joy they had once felt in returning home was overshadowed by the constant worry and the relentless progression of his illness.

For me, it was a time of deep sadness, not only because I was losing my father, but because I saw the toll it was taking on my mother as well. She had been his rock, standing by his side through every hospital stay, every treatment, and every setback. The weight of her worry and her grief was palpable, and as much as we tried to support her, it was clear that her heart was breaking as she watched the man she had spent her life with slowly slip away.

My own grief was complicated by the whirlwind of emotions I was already experiencing from the stresses of running the café. On top of the physical and emotional exhaustion that came with managing the business, I was now trying to navigate the overwhelming sorrow of watching my father's condition worsen. There were days when I felt utterly depleted, torn between the demands of my work and the desire to be there for my family. The café required my attention, but my heart was with my parents.

As the end drew near, we were all there, doing everything we could to make my dad's final days as peaceful as possible. It was a time filled with a strange mix of sorrow and love, as we gathered together to support each other and honour the man who had been such a central figure in our lives. We shared stories, memories, and quiet moments by his bedside, knowing that we were saying goodbye. His passing left a deep hole in all of us, a void that still lingers.

In many ways, this experience of losing my dad compounded the emotional toll of that period of my life. It felt like everything was happening at once trying to run a business, coping with the physical exhaustion from MS, and now, grieving the loss of a man who had been such a presence in my life. But as hard as it was, this time also reminded me of the importance of family, of the strength we draw from one another when life feels impossible to bear. We survived this heartbreaking chapter together, and that, more than anything, gave me the courage to keep going, even when the weight of the world felt too heavy to carry.

In the last three years of owning the café, I tried desperately to sell it. I knew that if I didn't let go, it would eventually break me. I needed to free myself, not only for the sake of my own sanity and health but for my family as well. The early death of my dad, to an auto-immune disease was no doubt playing on my mind. The business had become a burden that I could no longer carry, and I could feel it slowly consuming every aspect of my life. Every day I spent there felt like a battle, not just against the workload but against my own body's limitations. Yet, even as I fought to sell the café, I couldn't deny that there was a strange contradiction running through my experience.

MS & ME

On one hand, the exhaustion was relentless—physically, emotionally, and mentally, I was drained to the core. But on the other hand, there was a deep sense of fulfilment that came with it all. Despite the tears, the pain, and the overwhelming fatigue, there was something profoundly rewarding about the work I was doing. The connections I made with the people who walked through the doors, the sense of community the café fostered, and the knowledge that I was providing something meaningful to those around me—all of that brought me a strange kind of joy, even in the midst of the struggle.

*[**Health Insight**: Dr. Rebecca Lang, a psychologist specializing in chronic illness, notes that connection and community play a critical role in managing stress and maintaining mental health. "A sense of belonging can buffer the effects of physical challenges, providing emotional support that helps people cope with the demands of life," she explains.]*

It's a curious thing, how exhaustion and fulfilment can coexist like that, running side by side. They seem like opposites, and yet, in those years, they were inextricably linked. The café pushed me to my limits, but at the same time, it gave me a purpose that kept me going, even when I felt like I had nothing left to give.

Thankfully I wasn't also battling through monthly menstrual cramps. When I was teaching and into the mid 2000's I was often incapacitated every month. Like many women, I managed with paracetamol and hot water bottles. The best solution for me was having the Mirena Coil fitted, which, after a few months, stopped my periods entirely—a huge relief, especially as my periods had worsened my MS symptoms. By the time I had the device removed, after several painful attempts over the years, my doctor confirmed I had already gone through menopause, sparing me further discomfort. Absolute result!

MS & ME

(Expert Insight: "Menstrual pain and hormonal fluctuations can exacerbate symptoms of MS, such as fatigue, muscle spasms, and cognitive fog. The interplay between hormonal changes and MS inflammation highlights the importance of personalized care and symptom management during the menstrual cycle." – Dr. Rosalind Kalb, Neurologist and MS Specialist)

Around this time, I also experienced a significant shift in my MS treatment that brought with it a much-needed sense of relief. For years, I had been enduring the gruelling routine of deep muscle injections, which had become a dreaded part of my life. Every week, I braced myself for the thick needle to pierce through the muscles in the tops of my legs, alternating between each thigh, knowing that pain and discomfort would soon follow. These injections were not just physically painful—they were emotionally draining as well. Every time Simon administered the shot, I couldn't bear to look. The needle was so thick, and the pain so excruciating, that I needed a steady regimen of painkillers just to get through the day.

The process became a weekly ordeal, one that cast a shadow over my schedule. On injection days, I would prepare in advance, taking anti-inflammatory tablets and paracetamol, knowing that I was in for a day of flu-like symptoms and aching limbs. The fatigue would settle in, and I often found myself feeling completely drained, both physically and mentally. The injections, while necessary, were a constant reminder of my illness—a painful ritual that seemed to never end.

But then, in what felt like a turning point in my journey with MS, a new treatment emerged: a pill. I can't fully describe the sense of relief and gratitude I felt when I learned that I could finally say goodbye to those horrible injections. Instead of enduring the pain and side effects of deep muscle shots, I could now simply take a pill each day. It seemed almost too good to be true—a treatment that was not only easier to manage but would allow me to reclaim some of the time and energy I had lost to my old routine.

I remember the first day I took the pill, it felt like a weight had been lifted off my shoulders. I no longer had to brace myself for the weekly ordeal of injections, no more painful stabs in my legs, no more days spent battling the side effects. The simplicity of swallowing a pill each morning felt almost luxurious after what I had endured for so long. It was as if a part of my life had been restored to me, and I was incredibly grateful for this advancement in treatment.

This change in my medication didn't just relieve me physically—it had a profound impact on my overall well-being. Without the weekly cycle of pain and discomfort, I felt lighter, freer, and more capable of focusing on other aspects of my life. The pill represented more than just an easier treatment option; it was a symbol of progress, of hope, and of the possibility that things could get better.

I was able to reclaim my days, no longer tethered to the clock waiting for the inevitable pain. Instead, I could move forward with a renewed sense of gratitude, knowing that modern medicine had given me a reprieve from what felt like a never-ending battle with those injections. And for that, I was truly thankful.

Chapter 8

The Dawn of a New Beginning

After nearly seven punishing yet transformative years, we finally sold the café in December of 2018. It was a moment that felt both monumental and surreal—a mixture of relief, pride, and bittersweet emotion. The café had been my life for so long, consuming every ounce of my energy and attention, and the idea of stepping away from it was both exciting and daunting. I had poured so much of myself into that business, from its chaotic beginnings to its eventual success, and the day we signed the papers felt like the closing of a significant chapter.

The sale itself marked the end of an era, but it was also a beginning for the new owner, someone who saw the same potential and charm in the café that I had when I first envisioned it. I felt a sense of satisfaction in knowing that the café would continue on, thriving under new leadership, rather than fading into memory. And to my delight, the new owner has welcomed us with open arms whenever we return to visit Bristol. Each time we walk through those familiar doors, it's like stepping back into a part of my history, yet now I get to experience it as a customer, not the one running the show. It's a strange but wonderful feeling, seeing the café bustling with life, knowing that its legacy is still unfolding.

What's even more fulfilling is seeing how the new owner has not just maintained the café, but taken it to new heights. He has injected fresh ideas and energy into the place, making his own mark on its evolution while preserving the essence of what made it special. It's a great achievement when I see it still busy, buzzing with the hum of conversations, and continuing to serve as a beloved cornerstone of the local community. The faces may have changed, and the menu may have evolved, but the heart of the café remains the same—a place where people gather, share stories, and find a moment of connection in their busy lives.

In contrast, my previous business, the conference centre, didn't afford me this same feeling of continuity. When that chapter ended, it felt final, as though everything we had built was locked away in the past, never to be revisited. The café, however, continues to live on, and there's a deep sense of accomplishment in knowing that something I started is still thriving, even without me at the helm. Each time I see it bustling with activity, it feels like a validation of all the hard work, sacrifice, and sleepless nights that went into making it a success.

But selling the café wasn't just a business transaction—it was a moment of personal victory. It marked the culmination of years of struggle, but also the triumph of endurance. I had faced countless challenges—financial stress, physical exhaustion from managing my MS, and the emotional rollercoaster of keeping the business afloat—and yet, I had made it through. Letting go of the café, despite my personal challenges, wasn't easy, but knowing it's in good hands has given me a sense of closure and pride that I carry with me to this day.

Visiting the café now feels like returning to a part of myself. I walk through those doors with the memories of the countless hours spent behind the counter, the laughter shared with my staff, and the relationships built with regular customers who became part of the café's extended family. I watch as the new owner adds his own layers to the story, and I can't help but smile, knowing that I was the one who laid the foundation.

Selling the café allowed me to close a chapter, yes—but it also let me pass the torch, and there's something incredibly fulfilling about watching that torch burn brightly in someone else's hands. It's a legacy I never got to experience with my conference centre, which faded into the past when I stepped away. But here, with the café, I get to witness its ongoing journey, and that is a truly unique and rewarding experience.

Every time I see the café thriving, still held in high regard by the local community, it reaffirms that all those long days and sleepless nights were worth it. The café's continued success is more than just a business achievement—it's a testament to resilience, community, and the power of creating something that outlives you. I may no longer be behind the counter, but a piece of me will always remain within those walls, watching as the café continues to evolve, serve, and bring people together. And in that, I find not just satisfaction, but joy.

As hard as they were, I wouldn't trade those years for anything. They taught me resilience, strength, and the importance of knowing when to let go. While the café drained me, it also enriched my life in ways that are hard to put into words. And although I eventually had to step away for the sake of my health and my family, the lessons I learned during that time remain with me, a testament to the power of perseverance, even in the face of overwhelming adversity.

Chapter 9

A Time for A New Beginning

Here I was, for the first time in my life, with no job, no business, and no immediate need to chase a weekly wage. It was an entirely unfamiliar feeling—one I had never experienced before. Even during the few times I had taken a step back from work, like the 11 weeks of maternity leave when we had our first child, I had still been tethered to responsibilities. And even during school holidays when I was teaching, my mind was always preoccupied with lesson planning and preparation for the new term. But now, for the first time, there was no deadline looming, no pressing tasks, no schedules to manage. It was a strange, almost unsettling sensation, and it took a lot of getting used to.

At first, I felt adrift, almost jumpy, as though I had lost my sense of self, my identity. After years of always being 'on'—running businesses, raising children, working through endless to-do lists—suddenly having time on my hands was disorienting. I found myself at a bit of a crossroads, unsure of who I was without a business to run or a job to go to each day. The café, which had been such a big part of my life for nearly seven years, was no longer mine. The children were grown up, each heading off on their own adventures. Our middle son had set off for an exciting journey to Australia, a whole world away, while our eldest had settled just down the road, living with my mother, his grandmother. I looked around and realized the life I had built, the one that had consumed so much of my time and energy, had shifted into something quieter and less demanding.

MS & ME

I had all this newfound time, but the question lingered—what could I do with it? What would fill this new chapter of my life? I had spent so many years defining myself through work, through the businesses I built, and the roles I played, that without them, I felt a bit lost. I knew I couldn't just sit still, but I didn't want to rush into something that wasn't right for me either. So I started to think about what I truly wanted, what had always been simmering in the back of my mind. The answer wasn't immediately clear, but one thing I did know—despite the humour I now see in it—I didn't want to open another café!

What I did know was that I had a deep desire to help others. The idea of returning to teaching crossed my mind more than once. It had always been a profession I was passionate about, and I knew how much I loved connecting with students and helping them grow. But I also knew the realities of teaching—it's not just a job, it's a lifestyle, and one that demands everything from you. I knew myself well enough to know that if I went back to teaching, I would pour myself into it with such intensity that I would likely burn out. My personality is such that I always give 110%, and I realized that teaching would take more from me than I had left to give.

And then, right on cue, as if by some divine intervention, serendipity stepped in, as it so often does in my life. I've always been a strong believer that everything happens for a reason, and this time was no different. One day, while browsing online, I stumbled across a promotion for an all-women coaching certification program. Something about it immediately struck a chord deep within me. It was as though the universe had heard my inner question, "What's next?" and answered it in the form of this course. I felt an instant connection to the idea, and I knew, without hesitation, that this was my new path.

MS & ME

Coaching had always been something that resonated with me. I love helping people, mentoring them, and offering guidance. Throughout my life, I had accumulated a wealth of personal and professional experiences, and the thought of using that knowledge to support others was incredibly appealing. This course felt like it was made for me—a chance to take everything I had learned and pass it on to others who might need a helping hand, just as I had needed one at various points in my own journey.

The decision to undertake the training wasn't without its challenges, though. The coaching certification course was quite costly, and I hesitated for a moment, weighing the investment against the uncertainty of my new venture. But in my heart, I knew that this was the right move. It was something that would not only give me purpose but also bring me joy. I needed a new project, something to ignite that fire in me again, and this coaching program was exactly what I had been searching for, even before I knew it existed.

And so, I took the plunge. I signed up for the course, feeling a renewed sense of purpose. It was exciting to have a goal again, to feel that buzz of anticipation and challenge. I was embarking on something that was not only meaningful but deeply aligned with who I am and what I value. This was more than just a new career—it was a new reason to be, a new way to contribute and to make a difference in the lives of others.

Looking back, I realize how important that moment of transition was for me. It wasn't just about finding a job or filling the time—it was about rediscovering myself, redefining my purpose, and stepping into a new chapter with confidence and clarity. The coaching certification wasn't just a course—it was the key to unlocking a new version of me, one that I am excited to continue exploring.

In late 2019, I found myself in a period of deep reflection. It had been a year since I sold the café, and I spent much of that time rediscovering myself, figuring out what came next. My mother had moved up to Scotland, and Simon and I were planning to follow, waiting on a redundancy package from his employer to make the transition smoother. The redundancy package never came but arrived in its place was a global pandemic.

Just before the onset of covid 19 I found myself enduring a series of traumatic dental appointments, where I had to have several of my upper back teeth removed. It was a hard reminder of the importance of the vitamin D I'd never been told to take, a lesson learned too late. Just as I was processing that, the global pandemic hit, bringing even more uncertainty into our lives. In hindsight, I'm incredibly grateful that I wasn't among the many who had to suffer unbearable dental pain during such a difficult and chaotic time.

For me, the world coming to a standstill during the pandemic actually worked in my favour. The slower pace of life gave me the space I needed to focus on earning my Coaching certification. While many struggled, I was fortunate enough to have this opportunity to use that time productively. Looking back, I feel incredibly lucky for how things unfolded. The other positive I took from that awful time was it finally knocked my cigarette smoking habit on the head after a year of stopping and starting, sometimes for years at a time, the fear of weak lungs finally cracked it and I have now stopped forever.

I had long been drawn to practices that offered deeper insight into the mind-body connection—techniques that went beyond traditional approaches and allowed me to find balance in moments of stress and clarity when making difficult decisions. Meditation and relaxation had been key tools for me, particularly during the most stressful periods of my business life, and I often turned to these techniques when I needed to calm my mind and regain focus. They were not just coping mechanisms; they were pathways to finding inner strength and alignment in a world that often felt chaotic.

A few years earlier, while running the café, I had even negotiated some time off to pursue something I had been curious about for years: an NLP (Neuro-Linguistic Programming) Practitioner course. It was a transformative experience. NLP opened up new ways of understanding the power of language and thought patterns in shaping our reality. It gave me tangible tools for reframing challenges, both in business and in my personal life. That course planted seeds of deeper awareness, seeds that would eventually grow into a full-blown passion for helping others harness their own inner power.

What has always fascinated me is how these alternative therapies—meditation, NLP, relaxation techniques, and more—exist alongside conventional medicine. I firmly believe that there is a vast and necessary space for these more mystical approaches, a space where science and spirit intersect. Understanding the intricate relationship between the mind and the body has stirred something within me for as long as I can remember. It feels as though, at our core, we are capable of so much more than we realize. Our minds hold immense power over our physical bodies, and I have always believed that this connection is key to achieving well-being.

During my coaching training, I went through the program myself, and this experience was transformative in so many ways. It helped me truly understand my emotions, build resilience, and reflect on my relationships and life choices. For most people, coaching brings to the surface those late-night worries we've ruminated over but never fully addressed. It gives you the tools to explore and untangle long-held issues.

One of the most valuable lessons I learned was recognizing the triggers that send me into a downward spiral and, more importantly, how to manage them. I became aware of the ways I had been living up to the expectations of others—following cultural norms or societal standards that didn't necessarily serve my growth or well-being as a whole person. I now put my own well-being at the centre. I have regular Thai massages and I take daily exercise. I spend time doing things that I enjoy and I meditate most days.

While I had a superficial understanding of myself before, this deep dive into coaching gave me the insights I had been missing. It left me wishing I had discovered these truths earlier in life, as they've profoundly changed the way I approach both challenges and opportunities. The clarity I gained has been invaluable, and I now feel empowered to live more authentically, with greater self-awareness and purpose.

This belief in the potential of the mind, in our ability to influence our health and our lives through our thoughts, has been a quiet force guiding me for years, brought to a more conscious level since my coaching training. I believe that we have far more control over our physical and mental well-being than we give ourselves credit for. It's not just the medications that have sustained me through my struggles with MS, though I am grateful for the advances in pharmaceuticals that have eased my journey. It's also been this deep-seated belief in the power of the mind, the conviction that we can influence our own health, that has carried me through the toughest of times.

But these beliefs raise their own questions—questions that have lingered in my mind for years. If I truly believe in the power of the mind, in our ability to shape our health and lives, then why am I not 100% well? Why, after striving so hard to live in alignment with these principles, do I still face challenges with my health? It's a paradox I grapple with, and one that has pushed me to reflect more deeply on the complexities of the human experience.

I've come to believe that the answer lies not in a lack of faith in these practices, but in the fact that life is far more nuanced than we often care to admit. Yes, I believe wholeheartedly that the mind and body are deeply interconnected, and that how we live, think, and engage with the world has a profound impact on our health. But I also recognize that we are not immune to the random and uncontrollable elements of existence—the genetic predispositions, the environmental factors, the sheer unpredictability of life. The millions-to-one chance that any of us became who we are is a testament to how much we don't fully understand.

And perhaps that is part of the lesson. Maybe it's not about achieving perfect health or absolute control over our lives. Maybe it's about striving for balance, for deeper understanding, and for peace with the unknown. I've come to see that my journey has been less about eliminating illness or struggle, and more about embracing the tools and beliefs that help me navigate them. It's about using meditation, relaxation, and coaching not just to fix problems, but to approach life with more resilience, compassion, and curiosity.

I've realized that the act of striving itself—striving for wellness, for understanding, for growth—is where the real transformation lies. It's about being open to the possibilities, about believing in our capacity for healing while also accepting that we can't control everything. The power of the mind isn't in eliminating all struggle; it's in how we face that struggle, how we rise in the face of adversity, and how we continually search for ways to live our best lives, even when the odds feel stacked against us.

The gut-to-mind connection has, in my experience, had a profound impact on my overall health and well-being. Understanding how closely our digestive health is tied to our mental clarity, mood, and physical resilience has been a game-changer for me. I make a conscious effort to follow a very healthy diet, especially when it comes to my main meals. I prioritize whole, nutrient-dense foods, and most of what I eat is made from scratch, ensuring that I know exactly what is going into my body. Fresh vegetables, lean proteins, and healthy fats are staples in my kitchen, and I truly believe this approach has made a significant difference in how I feel, both physically and mentally. I nearly always avoid bread and as many wheat products as possible and when I do eat regular pasta and rice, I choose wholewheat or gluten-free varieties. I still have echoes back to the private consultant who recommended me to the Stone Age Diet, I believe it's now known as the Paleo Diet. For someone with more willpower than me, I would fully recommend this!

That said, I'm not going to pretend that I'm a perfect example of dietary restraint. I absolutely indulge in my cravings for chocolate or crisps from time to time! Life, after all, is about balance, and I don't believe in depriving myself completely. Instead, I remind myself that by maintaining a predominantly good gut-health-focused diet, I can afford the occasional treatment without repercussions. I supplement my meals with vitamins, probiotics, and Omega Balance oil that further support my gut health, reinforcing the idea that the overall picture of my health is positive and balanced. This approach allows me to enjoy those little indulgences, knowing that the foundation of my diet is solid and supportive of my long-term health. For me, it's all about keeping things in harmony—nourishing my body while allowing room for life's small pleasures.

So, while I may not be 100% well all the time, and while I continue to strive for greater health, I know that these beliefs have sustained me, shaped me, and carried me through some of the most difficult times in my life. And I truly believe they can do the same for others. This understanding, this passion for helping others discover the potential within themselves, is what has led me to this path of coaching, mentoring, and guiding others toward their own healing journeys. For me, It's about more than just health—it's about finding meaning, balance, and strength in the journey itself.

I was talking to a young woman recently who received a diagnosis of MS around a similar age to me she firmly believes, as I do, that the diagnosis has led her to a much healthier way of being. It's almost as though we have been afforded a wake-up call. Maybe we can be grateful for the new health-conscious ways of living the diagnosis has brought to our lives!

Chapter 10

Over to You

First, let me thank you for joining me on this journey. Writing this book has been both cathartic and fulfilling, but knowing it might help you find strength, joy, and purpose in your life brings me the greatest satisfaction. Now, let's turn the focus to you.

How can you start implementing changes, big or small, that will lead to a happier, healthier, and more fulfilling life? Here are practical steps, expert-backed advice, and personal insights to guide you.

Step 1: Start Small, Stay Consistent

When it comes to transforming your health and mindset, small changes done consistently over time lead to big results. You don't need to overhaul your life overnight—just pick one area to focus on and start there.

- **Actionable Tip:** Begin by creating one small daily habit that supports your health. For example:
    - Commit to drinking a glass of water first thing in the morning to hydrate your body.
    - Spend five minutes stretching to wake up your muscles and joints.
    - Go for a short walk in the fresh air—nature is a proven mood booster.

[Expert Validation]: Dr. James Lacey, a behavioral psychologist, emphasizes the importance of "micro-habits." He explains,

"Focusing on small, manageable goals builds momentum and helps cement long-term changes. These small wins lead to big victories."

Step 2: Develop Your Morning and Evening Rituals

How you start and end your day sets the tone for everything in between. Simple morning and evening rituals can ground you, reduce stress, and help you feel more in control.

- **Morning Ritual Ideas:**
    - **Gratitude Exercise:** Before getting out of bed, think of three things you're grateful for. This shifts your mindset toward positivity.
    - **Mindful Movement:** Try light yoga, breathing exercises, or even gentle tai chi.
    - **Fuel Your Day:** Have a balanced breakfast that includes protein, healthy fats, and fiber to stabilize your energy levels.

- **Evening Ritual Ideas:**
    - **Reflection Time:** Keep a gratitude journal by your bed. Write down three positive moments from your day.
    - **Unplug:** Turn off screens at least an hour before bed. Read a book, meditate, or enjoy some quiet time instead.
    - **Relaxation Techniques:** Practice deep breathing or listen to calming music to signal to your body that it's time to unwind.

[Personal Insight]: *When I began incorporating mindful mornings, my entire day seemed brighter. Even just taking a moment to breathe deeply or listen to a favorite song gave me the clarity and energy to face challenges.*

Step 3: Move for Joy

Exercise often feels like a chore, but when you find ways to move that genuinely bring you joy, it becomes something to look forward to.

- **Actionable Tip:** Experiment with different types of movement until you find what excites you. It might be dancing, swimming, hiking, or even gardening.
- **Keep it Social:** Invite friends or family to join you. It's easier to stay motivated when you're doing something fun together.

[Expert Validation]*: Studies show that exercise doesn't just strengthen your body—it boosts endorphins, reduces inflammation, and enhances mental clarity. Find what moves you, literally and emotionally!*

Step 4: Embrace the Power of Rest

Rest is not a luxury—it's a necessity, especially when managing health challenges. Adequate sleep and intentional downtime are critical for your mental and physical well-being.

- **Actionable Tip: Prioritize Quality Sleep**
    - Create a sleep-friendly environment: keep your bedroom cool, dark, and quiet.
    - If you work from home, where possible do not bring the office to your bedroom

- Look in to Feng Shui for your bedroom (at least)
- Establish a consistent bedtime routine, going to bed and waking up at the same time each day.
- Avoid caffeine or heavy meals in the evening, as they can interfere with restful sleep.

[Expert Validation]: Dr. Anna Price, a sleep researcher, emphasizes that restorative sleep is vital for people managing chronic conditions. "Sleep allows the body to repair itself, regulate inflammation, and improve cognitive function," she says.

Step 5: Nourish Your Body with Intention

Diet plays a significant role in how you feel day-to-day, especially when dealing with autoimmune conditions like MS. While there's no one-size-fits-all approach, adopting a balanced and anti-inflammatory diet can support your overall health.

- **Actionable Tip: Focus on Whole Foods**
    - Incorporate fresh vegetables, lean proteins, healthy fats (like avocado and nuts), and whole grains into your meals.
    - Experiment with anti-inflammatory spices like turmeric and ginger, which can help reduce inflammation and promote healing.
    - Limit processed foods, sugar, and refined carbohydrates—they may contribute to inflammation and energy crashes.
- **Gut Health is Key**:
    - Include probiotic-rich foods like yogurt, kimchi, or sauerkraut.

- Add prebiotics like bananas, oats, and asparagus to feed your gut's good bacteria.

[Personal Insight]: *I've made small but impactful changes to my diet over the years—opting for homemade meals, avoiding heavy processed foods, and focusing on gut-friendly options. It's not about perfection but balance. And yes, I still enjoy chocolate from time to time!*

Step 6: Manage Stress with Practical Tools

Stress is inevitable, but how you respond to it can make a world of difference. Chronic stress can exacerbate health issues, so building a stress-management toolkit is essential.

- **Actionable Tip: Discover What Works for You**
    - **Meditation:** Even five minutes of mindfulness or guided meditation can calm your mind and reset your perspective.
    - **Breathing Exercises:** Try the 4-7-8 technique: inhale for four counts, hold for seven, and exhale for eight.
    - **Creative Outlets:** Expressing yourself through art, writing, or music can be both therapeutic and joyful.
    - **Music is therapy**

[Expert Validation]: *Dr. Louise Carter, a stress management expert, states, "Stress amplifies inflammation and can trigger flare-ups in autoimmune conditions. Learning to manage it effectively improves both physical and mental health."*

Step 7: Build Your Support Network

You don't have to do this alone. Surround yourself with people who lift you up and support your journey.

- **Actionable Tip: Strengthen Relationships**
    - Reach out to friends or family who make you feel seen and valued.
    - Consider joining a support group for people with similar health challenges—it's powerful to connect with those who truly understand your experiences.
- **Seek Professional Support:**
    - A life coach, therapist, or counselor can provide guidance tailored to your goals and struggles.
    - Don't hesitate to consult with medical professionals regularly to ensure your treatments and strategies are optimized.

[Personal Insight]: My own journey would have been far lonelier without the support of my family, friends, and fellow MS warriors. They've been my cheerleaders, and I hope this book can be one of yours. Join my Women's Facebook group (see below).

Step 8: Take Ownership of Your Healthcare

Empowering yourself as an active participant in your health journey is transformative. Partnering with your healthcare providers and advocating for your needs can lead to better outcomes.

- **Actionable Tip: Educate Yourself**
    - Learn as much as you can about your condition. Knowledge is power, and being informed allows you to make choices with confidence.

- o   Stay updated on the latest research and treatment options. Follow reputable medical organizations or MS-focused resources.
- **Build a Collaborative Relationship with Your Doctor**
  - o   Prepare questions for your appointments to ensure you get the answers you need.
  - o   Share your goals and concerns openly, and don't be afraid to ask for second opinions when necessary.

[Expert Validation]: Dr. Emily Harrison, a neurologist, emphasizes, "Patients who are actively involved in their care tend to have better adherence to treatment plans and a greater sense of control over their health."

Step 9: Find Joy in Movement

Exercise isn't just about physical fitness—it's a cornerstone of emotional well-being, improved energy levels, and better symptom management.

- **Actionable Tip: Choose Activities You Enjoy**
  - o   If intense workouts aren't your thing, start with gentle yoga, tai chi, or even a daily walk in nature.
  - o   Explore adaptive fitness programs designed for those with mobility challenges, ensuring that exercise remains accessible.
- **Listen to Your Body:**
  - o   On days when fatigue or other symptoms are intense, it's okay to rest. Movement doesn't have to be rigid—flexibility is key.

MS & ME

[Personal Insight]: *My 50-squats-a-day challenge started as a fundraiser but became a game-changer for my core strength and energy. I didn't think I'd keep it up, but now it's one of my go-to rituals when I need a reset. Also dancing to your favourite music is a great mood changer.*

Step 10: Celebrate Your Wins

Big or small, every achievement deserves recognition. Life's journey isn't just about the destination but the steps we take along the way.

- **Actionable Tip: Create a "Win Journal"**
    - Write down one thing you're proud of each day. It could be as simple as getting out of bed on a tough morning or as significant as completing a major project.
- **Reflect on How Far You've Come:**
    - Periodically revisit old challenges you've overcome. Seeing your progress in black and white reinforces your resilience and inspires confidence.

[Expert Validation]: Dr. Chloe Martins, a psychologist, states, "Acknowledging achievements, no matter how small, helps reinforce positive behaviors and boosts self-esteem."

Step 11: Leverage Technology

In today's world, technology can be a powerful ally in managing your health and lifestyle.

- **Actionable Tip: Use Health Apps**
    - Track symptoms, manage medications, and set reminders for appointments or self-care practices using apps tailored to your needs.

Stay Connected:

- Virtual support groups and online communities provide a space to share your journey and learn from others.

[Personal Insight]: *Joining online forums for MS-related discussions helped me feel less alone. Hearing others' stories reminded me that we're all navigating this together, and there's strength in shared experiences.*

Step 12: Prioritize Mental Health

Living with a chronic condition often takes an emotional toll. Acknowledging and addressing your mental health is just as important as managing physical symptoms.

- **Actionable Tip: Seek Support**

    - Don't hesitate to reach out to a therapist or counselor if you're feeling overwhelmed, anxious, or depressed.
    - Look for specialists who understand chronic illness and its unique challenges.

- **Practice Emotional Resilience**

    - Incorporate mindfulness or meditation practices into your routine. These techniques help calm racing thoughts and build inner peace.
    - Journaling your feelings can also provide clarity and serve as an emotional outlet.

[Expert Validation]: *"Mental health is integral to overall well-being. Chronic conditions often blur the lines between physical and* *emotional challenges, making mental health care essential," says Dr. Amelia Parker, a licensed clinical psychologist.*

Step 13: Foster Strong Relationships

Isolation can creep in when dealing with health challenges, but nurturing your connections with others is vital for emotional health.

- **Actionable Tip: Share Your Journey**
    - Be open with close friends and family about your experiences. Sharing your feelings helps them understand how to support you better.

- **Set Healthy Boundaries**
    - While relationships are essential, it's also crucial to protect your energy. Learn to say no when you need to recharge and communicate your limits with kindness but firmness.

[Personal Insight]: My family has been my lifeline. Whether it's a listening ear or someone to lean on during flare-ups, knowing they're there keeps me grounded. At the same time, learning to say "no" to excessive commitments has been equally empowering.

Step 14: Plan for the Future with Hope

Thinking ahead doesn't mean dwelling on "what ifs." Instead, it's about creating a sense of control and preparedness that empowers you to live fully in the present.

- **Actionable Tip: Financial and Practical Planning**
    - Explore insurance options, retirement plans, and savings accounts that can support long-term health care or other needs.

- Have open conversations with loved ones about your wishes and any contingencies.
- **Set Life Goals**
  - Whether it's taking a dream vacation, starting a hobby, or mentoring others, let your goals reflect what truly matters to you.

[Expert Validation]: Financial adviser Angela Brooks states, "Planning for the future can be daunting but also freeing. It's a way to reclaim control over aspects of life that may feel unpredictable."

Step 15: Redefine Success

Success isn't one-size-fits-all—it's about aligning with what fulfills you personally, not living up to others' standards.

- **Actionable Tip: Create Your Own Metrics**
  - Define what success looks like for you today. It might be as simple as having the energy to enjoy a meal with friends or as ambitious as launching a new project.
- **Celebrate Growth Over Perfection**
  - It's okay if plans shift or goals evolve. What matters most is that you're moving forward at your own pace.

[Personal Insight]: For me, success isn't about chasing grandiose achievements anymore—it's about living a balanced, meaningful life. Writing this book, for instance, was a milestone that reminded me success can come in different forms.

Step 16: Understand the Bigger Picture

One of the most striking revelations about autoimmune diseases is how cultural factors play an outsized role in their prevalence, particularly among women. Dr. Gabor Maté, in an interview with Susie Moore, highlighted this stark reality:

"Women have 80% of autoimmune disease… It's not biological, it's not gendered. It's cultural."

This profound observation serves as both a wake-up call and a call to action. It underscores the importance of examining the societal pressures and expectations placed on women—the roles they're expected to fill, the emotions they're taught to suppress, and the relentless drive to care for others, often at the expense of their own well-being.

Step 17: Embrace Empowerment

Living with an autoimmune condition, or any chronic illness, doesn't mean surrendering to it. It means learning how to stand tall in the face of challenges, rewrite the narrative, and reclaim your power.

- **Actionable Tip: Advocate for Yourself**
    - Speak up in medical appointments; you are the expert on your body. Don't be afraid to ask questions or seek second opinions if necessary.
    - Educate yourself about your condition. The more you know, the more effectively you can make decisions that align with your values and goals.
- **Be an Ally to Others**
    - Sharing your story can inspire others who may be struggling silently. By being open and honest, you create a ripple effect of understanding and support.

[Personal Reflection]: For years, I carried the weight of trying to be everything to everyone. It took time (and a lot of self-coaching!)

to realize that my value isn't tied to how much I do for others. My worth lies in who I am, not what I produce.

Step 18: Create Community

The journey of managing health challenges is made easier with a strong support system. Building connections with others who share similar experiences can provide immense comfort and guidance.

- **Actionable Tip: Join Support Networks**
    - Whether it's an online forum, a local group, or a one-on-one connection, finding a space to share your thoughts and learn from others can be transformative.

- **Celebrate Collective Wins**
    - When someone in your community achieves a milestone—whether it's starting a new treatment or simply having a good day—celebrate it together. These shared moments of joy create bonds that uplift everyone.

[Expert Validation]: *Dr. Sarah Watson, a community health advocate, states, "The power of connection cannot be overstated. Feeling seen, heard, and understood is one of the most healing experiences anyone can have."*

Closing Thoughts

As you close this chapter and look ahead to the next phase of your journey, remember that the most important thing you can do is honor yourself—your needs, your dreams, and your well-being.

- Find strength in knowing you're not alone.
- Cultivate joy in the small moments.

    Trust in your capacity to adapt and grow.

- Journal your progress and reflect for clarity

And most importantly, live fully—because this life, with all its twists and turns, is still a gift.

Step 19: Pay It Forward

If you've found value in this book, I ask you to take a few moments to share your thoughts. Your feedback can inspire others who might need this guidance and encouragement.

Please take a couple of minutes to post a review.

Step 20: Stay Connected

If this book has resonated with you and you'd like to continue your journey toward greater health and fulfilment, I invite you to join me in exploring more tools, tips, and inspiration.

- **Visit My Website:** Discover journals, resources, and more at www.lmcpublications.com.

- **Join the Community:** For women seeking connection, empowerment, and a safe space to share their journeys, check out my LauraMc Coaching Facebook group. Together, we can support one another as we navigate life's challenges and celebrate its victories.

MS & ME

Dedication

This book is dedicated to everyone who has faced the challenges of autoimmune diseases with courage, resilience, and grace. May this book inspire hope, healing, and empowerment.

As you finish this book and take your next steps, I hope you carry with you the belief that you are capable of creating a fulfilling, meaningful life. While challenges are inevitable, how you meet them defines the story you tell about yourself. Be proud of your journey, honor your resilience, and never stop seeking the light within you.

Thank you for trusting me to share this part of your path. It has been my honor to walk with you. 🩶

Love
Laura

MS & ME

Thank You for Reading

Your honest review helps others discover this book and allows me to continue sharing resources that inspire and support those living with MS.

Looking for more tools to support your journey? Don't forget to check out my **12-Month MS Journal**, designed to help you track your progress, mindset, and well-being.

Simply scan the QR code below or visit my website to share your thoughts and explore more resources:

🌐 **Visit:** www.lmcpublications.com

Thank you for your support and for being part of this journey. Your voice truly matters!

With gratitude,
Laura Lamont

Printed in Great Britain
by Amazon